Further praise for *The Roadmap to 100*

"More and more people are living well into their eighties and nineties today and they are continuing to thrive and participate fully in life. Renowned physician and aging _____ m the Stanford Medical School makes _____ umatically impact our own lifelong hea_____ ed exercise. He draws on cutting edge _____ veaker as the decades pass, not necessarily due to aging, but rather because we don't challenge our bodies enough. *The Roadmap to 100* shows how staying engaged cuts across all fields—exercising, socializing, keeping sexuality alive—can prolong your life for many decades. This is a fantastic book and Bortz is a true trailblazer."

—Ken Dychtwald, Ph.D., author of
The Age Wave and *A New Purpose:*
Redefining Money, Family, Work, Retirement, and Success

"At 80 years young, Doctor Walter Bortz brings an energy to his work that exceeds most 20 year olds. He challenges us with an uplifting message: we are each ultimately responsible for our own health, and that by remaining fully engaged—in our communities, in physical fitness, by maintaining our intellect and being creative—we can extend our lives and make them worth living."

—Jim Collins, author of *Good to Great*

"Unlike the generalizations with which doctors usually instruct their patients, this book outlines in clear, concise prose what we can do to remain fully functional as we age. Moreover, it explains exactly how the interventions recommended work to preserve health and competence. The book is a welcome aid to helping people live better as well as longer."

—Marianne Legato, author of *Why Men Die First*

"With his enthusiasm and insight, Walter Bortz makes us want to go further and explore all the options of aging. *The Roadmap to 100* is a spirited romp through the process of gaining wisdom and pleasure as we continue on and on."

—Bonnie Matheson, author of *Ahead of the Curve*

"Here is a fast paced and lively guide on how to live longer. Wally Bortz's clear and direct message emphasizes the importance of action, motion, and engagement in maintaining 'vim and vigor'."

—Seth Landefeld, M.D., Professor of Medicine,
Chief, Division of Geriatrics,
University of California at San Francisco

"Ever since I learned that Jeanne Calment said at 120 she had only one wrinkle, and she was sitting on it, I figured that humor must be the key to longevity. Since then I met Walter M. Bortz—marathoner, thinker, and former head of the American Geriatrics Association. No one has been a more avid gatherer and popularizer of data on the importance of exercise to the project of happiness and longevity. But Bortz's vision extends further, to a whole new medicine based on empowerment and prevention, and informed by evolution and energy science. Bortz's vision is contagious, and I'm a subscriber!"

—Dorion Sagan, author of *Biospheres*

"With longevity becoming the new norm, we can use all the help we can get from the experts to help us along."

—Edgar Mitchell, Sc.D. Founder of the Institute
of Noetic Sciences; Astronaut Apollo 14.

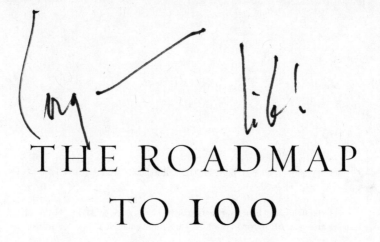

THE ROADMAP
TO 100

The Breakthrough Science of

Living a Long and Healthy Life

WALTER M. BORTZ II, M.D.

RANDALL STICKROD

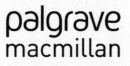
palgrave
macmillan

THE ROADMAP TO 100
Copyright © Walter M. Bortz II, MD, and Randall Stickrod, 2010.
All rights reserved.

First published in hardcover in 2010 by PALGRAVE MACMILLAN® in the US—
a division of St. Martin's Press LLC, 175 Fifth Avenue, New York, NY 10010.

Where this book is distributed in the UK, Europe and the rest of the world, this is by
Palgrave Macmillan, a division of Macmillan Publishers Limited, registered in England,
company number 785998, of Houndmills, Basingstoke, Hampshire RG21 6XS.

Palgrave Macmillan is the global academic imprint of the above companies and has
companies and representatives throughout the world.

Palgrave® and Macmillan® are registered trademarks in the United States, the United
Kingdom, Europe and other countries.

ISBN: 978-0-230-11205-6

Library of Congress Cataloging-in-Publication Data

Bortz, Walter M.
   The roadmap to 100 : the breakthrough science of living a long and healthy life /
Walter Bortz and Randall Stickrod.
      p.   cm.
   Includes bibliographical references and index.
   ISBN 978-0-230-10068-8 (hardback)
   (paperback ISBN 978-0-230-11205-6)
   1. Longevity. 2. Health. 3. Aging—Prevention. I. Stickrod, Randall.
II. Title.   III. Title: Roadmap to one hundred.
RA776.75.B674   2010
613.2—dc22

                                                            2010000526

A catalogue record of the book is available from the British Library.

Design by Letra Libre

First PALGRAVE MACMILLAN paperback edition: September 2011

10 9 8 7 6 5 4 3 2 1

Printed in the United States of America.

To our families, present and future. To all of those on whose shoulders we have stood.

—*Walter M. Bortz II, M.D. and Randall Stickrod*

CONTENTS

THE ROADMAP
TO 100

INTRODUCTION

We live in a world divided by health. Any large city today probably has more gyms and health clubs than gas stations. We have bike lanes and urban hiking trails, the hallmarks of an active, aware population embracing fitness and robust health. And yet, our headlines blare out chilling warnings about the epidemic of obesity and the rampaging spread of type 2 diabetes, a disease that barely existed just two generations ago. Fitness scores among school-age children continue to drop precipitously. Fast food franchises seem to be everywhere, contrasting with the increasing presence of organic foods and farmers' markets. We are a population dangerously divided between the health conscious and the health averse.

Nearly every day we read a story about a new centenarian, the fastest-growing demographic category in the country. It seems a thrilling affirmation that we are still progressing, still evolving as a species, still the pinnacle of the evolutionary food chain. Masters of the universe further asserting our mastery by extending the very span of our lives. But in the same paper, there will be at least one story about our soaring health care costs, signs of a major national crisis. We are getting early warnings that our average life span may well decline in the next generation, the first such occurrence in the entire history of mankind.

The division between those who live long, productive lives with a real likelihood of achieving a full century, and those who merely progress deeper into the high-risk categories of medical statistics as they descend farther into middle age is increasing. What to make of all this?

Knowledge is power, it is said, and if knowledge can empower us to achieve and maintain our maximum health and enable us to live to our full potential, then we have truly accomplished something spectacular.

Yet too few are living anywhere close to their full potential. We all know the basics: Don't smoke. Don't drink too much. Eat your vegetables, and lay off the fast food. Exercise. The message becomes a mantra that is too easily ignored. We know you need more information in order to create a coherent and compelling message that can effectively cause you to modify your behavior. You need better answers: Not just what, but why? How? How much? How much should I exercise? Why should I lift weights if I'm not a bodybuilder? How much is too much? Why, exactly, should I avoid anything made with high-fructose corn syrup? We are accustomed to being told what we should or shouldn't do, but more often than not without the specifics of the reasons why. We need better, deeper, more detailed information.

Even many of our medical professionals are hard pressed to give the average person solid answers to questions like these. The typical medical school graduate is better trained to look for what's wrong with you than to shepherd you on a preventive path with specific goals of health, not to mention longevity. Imagine a routine physical exam where the patient asks the doctor these hard questions: What should I do to be as healthy as I possibly can? To live as long as I possibly can without loss of function? What kind of exercise should I do, how often, and how much? What should I eat? What shouldn't I eat? Should I take vitamins? Supplements? Is there anything I should stop doing because I'm now 70 years old?

One might get lucky. Some doctors are quite prepared to become your trusted advisor and guide you to all the best and most current information about health science. They are the exceptions, though. Medicine has been described as the newest science, and since medicine synthesizes biology, chemistry, and physics, it's no wonder that it has been a bit of a laggard. You don't have to look back too far to appreciate just how daunting the challenge has been. For instance, just a few decades ago, a patient who had suffered a heart attack was consigned to bed rest and almost total inactivity for weeks after the event. We now know that this is just about the worst thing you can do when recovering from a heart attack!

Medicine is problematic only to the extent that we let it be. As a culture we have become accustomed to turning to medicine and pharmaceuticals to make us well. Too many of us expect to be able to blithely defy all the advisories about healthy living and then turn to our doctor (or pharmacist) to fix the damage for us. In this respect, we have largely abdicated ownership of our health.

Who owns your health? You do! That admission is the first step toward blowing out those 100 candles on your milestone birthday cake.

The mission of this book is to present the case for living to 100 or more and living well all the while. We want you to avoid that long decline, the infirmities and frailties of later years, the degradations of helplessness and loss of independence. We are issuing a clarion call to reclaim ownership of our health, to learn to take responsibility for it and not rely blindly on medical technology to repair the damage we do to ourselves. The willingness to take responsibility for one's own health and well-being is the crucial first step; without that commitment all the other information here may well be irrelevant.

The roadmap to 100 passes through points that are all health related, a critical distinction that cannot be overstated. Longevity is neither an accident nor an isolated phenomenon. It is a product of specific healthy behaviors, a direct consequence of health maintenance. People who live to 100 are healthy people. They make better choices, choices that directly support the maintenance of healthy life processes and ward off the diseases that cut life short. Knowledge of these centenarian strategies is indeed power: the power to defy the default scenario of inevitable decline laid out by Mother Nature.

Various forecasts predict that by the middle of this century, as many as 6 million centenarians will be among us. The majority of them will be demonstrably healthy, functional, and largely independent. Many are expected to continue to be productive members of society, not simply retirees. The positive impact on our economy from having an elder cadre that contributes more than their social cost is exciting to anticipate, and unprecedented in world history.

Other forecasts predict a darker side, that the present trend toward obesity will increasingly become a global phenomenon, that type 2 diabetes will continue to spread with the "western diet" and ravage the world's population. Present estimates point to nearly 400 million people with diabetes worldwide by 2025, creating an insurmountable social burden as the cost of medical care continues to escalate, and the sick spend fewer years contributing as productive members of society. And the crisis will impact not just our own national health care costs but will have a global economic impact as well.

It is up to us to determine which of these scenarios will come to dominate the world we bequeath to future generations. Nobody wants to see the worst-case scenario—a downward spiral with immense social costs. An increasingly healthy population, in which people can expect to be productive members of society far longer than any previous time in our history, would be truly revolutionary, and worthy of what our species' potential has always promised.

CHAPTER 1

AGING, HEALTH, AND THE QUEST FOR LONGEVITY

THE CENTENARIAN IMPERATIVE

Growing old is a relatively recent phenomenon. Until the last century or two, the average life span was less than 30 years. The historical record on aging is so sparse that we have had little information about the aging process, and because so few people had the opportunity to achieve their full aging potential, we are just now learning what our potential life spans are. Prior to the agricultural revolution of 10,000 or so years ago, life was usually cut short by predation, injury, or starvation. The emergence of agriculture led to the formation of villages and cities; with people settling in close proximity, we saw the rise and spread of infectious diseases, which continued to inhibit average life spans. It wasn't until the twentieth century that average life expectancy began to rise appreciably, thanks to the medical successes curing infectious diseases, the widespread availability of food, and fewer hazards of daily life in civilized society. In fact, in the twentieth century alone, we have added approximately 30 years to the average life span, a near doubling over the previous millennia.

A century ago there were only a handful of centenarians on earth. By 1950 their numbers were estimated to be a few thousand. Today there are thought to be 340,000 centenarians worldwide, and it is estimated that that number will increase to 6 million by 2050. The highest concentrations of centenarians are projected to be in the United States and Japan. In 2009 there were approximately 100,000 in the United States and nearly 40,000 in Japan, but by mid-century those numbers are expected to grow to at least 600,000 in the United States and a full million in Japan, making centenarians the fastest-growing demographic, more than 20 times the overall rate of total population growth.

These impressive statistics underscore the viability of 100 as a reasonable objective, a longevity beacon that is demonstrably achievable. And yet we find ourselves in an era when the upward progression of expected life span is seriously threatened by an epidemic of lifestyle-based negative factors. Obesity and diabetes are the scourge of our times, a peculiar regression in a century of generally improving public health and longevity. We are increasingly becoming a bifurcated society, with one segment focused on health, fitness, and nutrition, and the other skewing our public health statistics in the negative direction. Probably the greatest challenge in public health policy today is to provide the education and motivation for the unhealthy to turn their lives around and adopt healthier—and hence more productive—lifestyles.

There is nothing special or magical—or particularly scientific—about the number 100, it should be noted. It is a convenient marker on our decimal-based number system, a "round" number in three digits, that just happens to be statistically significant in life-span studies. But it is a useful symbolic target. What we do know so far is that there seems to be a natural upper limit to the human life span, somewhere around 120 years. The oldest documented person was France's Mme. Jean Calment, who died in 1997 at the age of 122 (and who famously drank two glasses of port wine a day, made a hip-hop record at 121, and claimed to have "an enormous will to live and a good appetite, especially for chocolate").

Not long ago a newspaper item proclaimed the 115th birthday of Los Angeles resident Gertrude Baines and noted the irony in the fact that the world's oldest person would be found in the world's most youth-obsessed city. More remarkable than her age was the fact that, until she was 107, she lived independently and self-sufficiently. Reports of people achieving their 100th birthday are now becoming commonplace. There are now enough people in the United States who have reached an additional decade, 110 years of age, for us to coin a special term for them, "super-centenarians." At the time of this writing, 75 super-centenarians are being monitored by the Gerontology Research Group of Inglewood, California, and their ranks are slowly increasing.

It is as natural as breathing to want to extend life to its maximum limit. And yet who wants to live infirm, beset with frailty and loss of self-efficacy? Who wants to spend their last years—or decades—bedridden and hooked up to machines? It should be obvious that longevity and health are flip sides of the same coin. Longevity without health is not a desirable outcome for anyone. In fact it's not even an option. It is the convergence of the aging process and the quality of our health that determines our life span.

An extensive study by a Danish research group, covering 30 developed countries, now projects that of the babies born in these countries today, fully half should live to 100 or more. More importantly, these people are expected to encounter less disability and fewer functional limitations as they age, a consequence of presumed healthier lifestyles. The half that will not reach 100 will likely continue the other notable trend of our times, the increasing rate of obesity and diabetes that are tugging longevity statistics in the other direction.

Who wouldn't want to live to 100 or more, to have the longest possible life span? Not everyone, apparently. According to a survey by the

Pew Research Group, only 8 percent of Americans actually expressed a desire to live to 100. The reason is that most of us still associate that age with infirmity and a very low quality of life. The image invoked by a 100-year-old person is invariably one dominated by the things that a person can no longer do, of loss of independent living and degraded function. What is desirable about living that long if you can't do the things that seemed to make life worth living in the first place?

We believe that this view of late life is demonstrably wrong. One's later years are not fated to catastrophic decline and decrepitude, and we can now assert with the support of solid science that a great deal of the aging process is within our personal control. But first we have to understand just what the aging process is—and is not.

AGING IS NOT A DISEASE

A browse through the obituary pages of any major newspaper today reveals a subtle change that has taken place in the vernacular of dying over the last generation or two. It used to be commonplace, when almost anyone over the age of 60 succumbed, to attribute their death to "old age" or at least "natural causes." Today it is rare to see death reduced to such simple, non-clinical terms. If an 88-year-old's heart stops beating, it will likely be referred to as "cardiac failure," on the presumption that something went wrong, presumably the result of cardiac disease and not the programmed exhaustion of heart function, the predictable wear and tear of aging. Dying no longer requires disease as a handmaiden.

The urge to defy aging and its negative consequences seems as fundamental as the urge to procreate. That is understandable. What is not understandable is the notion that we can find a "cure" for aging and simply use a pill, an injection, or a surgical procedure as soon as medical science unlocks that secret. If aging were a disease, it's one that we were all born with and are destined to succumb to.

Aging is an inescapable reality, as immutable as the fundamental laws of physics. But its effects can be mitigated through conscious choices we make in everyday life. Aging does not have to imply infirmity, disease, frailty, or the inability to live full, productive, satisfying lives.

Our current remedial approach to aging is derived from the disease model of the medical profession. We look to potions, pills, medications. We look to gene therapies and radical surgeries. All of these approaches derive from the medical model that began with the French scientist Louis Pasteur in the mid-nineteenth century. From the time of the agricultural revolution until just a few decades ago, the primary threat to our health was infectious diseases: bubonic plague, smallpox, cholera, polio, tuberculosis, malaria, to name a few. Pasteur's discovery that the agents of these diseases were tiny microbes was a breakthrough that allowed us to combat them effectively. Ever since, medical science has been remarkably successful at finding remedies and preventive strategies for these diseases, and in many cases actually wiping them out. These successes have effectively entrenched the disease model as the de facto operating model of medicine for the past 150 years.

Surprisingly, aging has historically been poorly understood in the medical science community. Or perhaps not so surprisingly. Medicine can be considered in many ways our youngest science—physics, chemistry, and biology were established disciplines long before Pasteur and long before we had an accredited school of medicine with a science-based curriculum. The sheer complexity of living processes presents a daunting challenge, and requires not only a solid platform of the core sciences, but also a way of bringing them together to synthesize these disciplines into a new, emergent science of life. Aging has for too long been considered a process that is in opposition to living; and perhaps even more to the point, it is a process that has been largely shrouded in mystery.

TIME'S ARROW

Everything ages. It is the nature of our universe to change over time. Some 14 billion years from the Big Bang, time still ticks off its metrics, marking not just living things, but all matter. Even our fundamental particles—neutrons, electrons, protons—decay over time. Change is constant, everywhere, and inescapable. Without change, in fact, the concept of time would be meaningless. The arrow of time points in one direction only, an anomaly of physics, where everything else can go either forward or backward. Time, as a variable, frequently appears in most of the mathematical equations used to describe the physical world. Whether time flows backwards or forwards usually makes no difference in mathematics. But in our everyday world we never see time flowing backwards—from the present into the past. The fact that time is observed to flow inexorably only in one direction in real life is known as "time's arrow." The reason we experience time in only one direction, from past to present to future, is a consequence of the second law of thermodynamics, which is central to all life processes.

Thermodynamics is the science of energy production and exchange. Its laws govern everything associated with living and being alive, particularly our metabolic processes, those mechanisms of energy production and conversion that literally define what it means to be alive. The first law is often called the law of conservation of energy. It says that energy cannot be created or destroyed, that the amount of energy available in the universe is a constant. Einstein's famous equation, $E = mc^2$, can be thought of as part of this same concept, that energy and matter are interchangeable. The second law, simply stated, says that energy tends to spontaneously disperse. Entropy is a way of measuring that dispersal. Though the second law is the one we associate with the aging process, the first law is notable as the ironclad principle of all diet and weight loss systems—that weight loss happens only when the number of calories expended exceeds calorie intake, no matter what the source of calories.

The second law has become famous as the reason that such concepts as perpetual motion machines and "free energy" sources are impossible. It is the law from which the principle of entropy is derived. Entropy describes how things in nature tend toward increasing disorder, a scattering of available energy.

Our bodies age because, over time, things, including our internal structures, tend to become increasingly disordered. By analogy, we build things such as buildings, cars, and machines in orderly, systematic structures according to specific design criteria and with an investment of energy. But over time they tend to decay, to fall apart, and their components disperse. This is why, among other things, our skin may start out taut and smooth and over decades accrue wrinkles and begin to sag. Our DNA programs our structure, but entropy tends to work against the orderliness of our programmed form over time.

Living systems are "open" systems that continuously exchange matter and energy with their environment. When our cells replicate, they use our DNA as a blueprint to create new cells. Entropy is not just about the dispersal of energy, but about the loss of information in the process.

Entropy ensures that the process of cell replication is not perfect, that over time the organism is going to experience changes as the result of a subtle loss of information from one cycle to the next.

THE LIFE—AND DEATH—OF A CELL

Cells are the structural and functional units of living organisms, the "building blocks" of life. All of our life processes begin at the cellular level, and our health and wellness originates in our cells. The word *cell* comes from the Latin *cellula,* meaning "a small room," a designation given by the seventeenth-century polymath and inventor of the microscope, Robert Hooke, when he compared the cork cells he saw through his microscope to the small rooms monks lived in.

Mitochondria are the energy factories of the cells. They produce energy-rich molecules called adenosine triphosphates (ATPs). ATPs are produced in the mitochondria using the energy stored in food. Just as the chloroplasts in plants act as sugar factories for the supply of ordered molecules to the plant, the mitochondria in animals act to produce the ATP molecules as the energy supply for the processes of life. The conversion from food to energy molecules is a chemical reaction, fueled by oxygen. The reaction also produces free radicals as byproducts. These ionized molecules are highly reactive, and in turn create oxidative stress within the mitochondria. Oxidative stress leads to

mitochondrial mutations, a kind of vicious cycle in which enzymatic ab-
normalities are created, leading to further oxidative stress. This is what
signals the cumulative breakdown process we call "aging."

A number of changes occur to mitochondria during the aging
process. Tissues from elderly patients show a decrease in key enzymatic
activities. Large deletions in the mitochondrial genome can lead to high
levels of oxidative stress and trigger the neuronal death that leads to
Parkinson's disease. Hypothesized links between aging and oxidative
stress are not new and were proposed over 50 years ago; however, there
is much debate over whether mitochondrial changes are causes of aging
or merely characteristics of aging. Regardless, we know that to effectively deal with the effects of aging, it is necessary to understand mitochondrial processes.

Free radicals are a by-product of normal metabolism, but they also
come from smoking, pollution, toxins, and fried foods among other
things. Free-radical damage is associated with an increased risk of many
chronic diseases. Antioxidants such as vitamin C, carotenes, and vitamin E can reduce the damage caused by free radicals. Fortunately for
us, those antioxidants are commonplace components of a normal,
healthy diet.

Every cell at rest carries on its base activity. All of the cell's hundreds
to thousands of receptor sites—proteins in the cell walls—are continu-
ally scanning the environment for energetic cues, whether chemical,

thermal, mechanical, electrical, or magnetic, which initiate a repertoire of cellular reactions, both functional and structural. The genes listen in to this cueing, and turn on or turn off according to their programmatic function.

As you read this, millions of your cells are dying. Most of them are either superfluous or potentially harmful, so you're better off without them. In fact, your health depends on the judicious use of programmed cell death. The cells even come primed for self-destruction, equipped with the instructions and instruments. First, the cell shrinks and pulls away from its adjacent cells. Then, the surface of the cell begins to decompose, fragmenting and breaking away.

There is another kind of cell death, necrosis, that is unplanned. Necrosis can result from a traumatic injury, infection, or exposure to a toxic chemical. During necrosis, the cell's outer membrane loses its ability to control the flow of liquid into and out of the cell. The cell swells and ultimately bursts, releasing its contents into the surrounding tissue. Immune cells then flood the affected tissue, but the chemicals the cells use cause the area to become inflamed and sensitive. Burns from a hot stove are a commonplace example, with resulting redness and pain.

Many different kinds of injuries can cause cells to die via necrosis. It is what happens to heart cells during a heart attack, to cells in severely frostbitten fingers and toes, and to lung cells during a bout of pneumonia.

TELOMERES

Within our cells, our DNA molecules reside in our chromosomes, carrying the codes that define our nature. Each DNA strand is capped with telomeres, which cover the ends of the chromosome, much like the plastic caps on the ends of shoelaces protect the shoelace from unraveling. In the course of normal cell growth and replication, the telomeres are progressively shortened until they reach a built-in limit. At that point the cell can no longer divide (the process known as mitosis), and it will begin to die. The limit of the number of times a telomere can shrink is known as the Hayflick limit, after microbiologist Leonard Hayflick, who discovered the phenomenon.

The enzyme telomerase, which is produced both naturally and synthetically, has been found to inhibit the shortening of telomeres and hence has generated intense research activity to determine if it might be a way of extending life. The 2009 Nobel Prize in medicine was awarded to researchers doing pioneering work in this very area. Unfortunately, telomerase is also associated with cancer cells and their unregulated growth. A great deal of research and discovery remains to be done in this area.

DEFINING HEALTH

We speak of health in casual language, as if its meaning is universally understood. But to many, it is merely the absence of disease, whereas there is another large part of the population that would consider their health compromised if they fell below a certain level of fitness. What we know for certain is that health and longevity are intertwined. No examination of longevity can be carried on without a thorough understanding of health: its definition, its components, and what its gradations mean.

> Health is a state of complete physical, mental, and social well-being and not merely the absence of disease or infirmity.

This definition, adopted by the World Health Organization at its founding in 1946, is surprisingly still considered controversial. We find it laudable in its sweep and intent, but vague and subjective. One person's notion of what constitutes "well-being" might vary wildly with another's. Health clearly must be framed in terms of our potential as living organisms. We are the product of millions of years of evolution, of Darwinian adaptation and refinement. The question we must ask is, Are we functioning as our design has encoded us to? When every component functions optimally—and *function* is surely the key verb—then we are indisputably in a state of optimal health.

This assertion may beg the question of just what is our potential, anyway? Health ought to be seen in terms of how close we are to the limits of what we might potentially be. We can better understand our potential—and its limiting factors—by analyzing the biological determinants of health.

THE DETERMINANTS OF HEALTH

It is useful to think of health in terms of four basic factors that, taken together, determine the state of our health. The metaphor of car health helps to illustrate this. The life of a car depends on four elements: design, accidents, maintenance, and aging. If the car has design flaws, is involved in a major accident, or is poorly maintained, it will not have the chance to grow old. The same four categories apply to the human organism, but are more appropriately designated genes, external factors, internal factors, and aging. These four factors, occurring in innumerable combinations and chronologies, account for the totality of the human health experience, both individual and collective. Hypothetically, if the first three of these four factors could be stabilized through a perfect design or gene set, if there were no accidents or external disruptions, and if there were ideal maintenance and balanced internal dynamics, then we would have the opportunity to die of natural causes at the limit of our potential.

THE GENE FACTOR

It is popularly thought that genes, our family heritage, are the key factors behind our chances for an exceptionally long life. This is part of a broader misunderstanding about genes.

There is a widespread misconception that genes are fixed agents of determinism that largely regulate who we are and what we will become. "It's in your genes" carries a familiar fatalism. This tends to give the impression that we are fated for certain outcomes, that much of what befalls us is beyond our control.

There are many things wrong with this interpretation. Considering how well we now know the composition and biochemistry of genes, these misconceptions are hard to justify.

The acclaim accompanying the Human Genome Project gave the unwarranted impression that we were on the threshold of being able to fully decode our genetically driven life processes. This assumption has proved to be categorically false and misleading, much to the detriment of public awareness of gene science. In the public mind there persists a notion that specific genes control specific functions and determine specific health outcomes, like the onset of a great many diseases as well as our life span.

First, genes must be "expressed." What that means is that they are like switches that must be turned on in order to perform their designated functions. An even better way to think about it is to think of genes as functioning like a dimmer switch, with variable responsivity, not just a simple on-off capability. Second, genes typically act in concert, in groups or even networks.

We now know a critical dimension of the gene story: Genes are rarely intended to function independently. They work in coordinated ensembles, which in turn are closely matched with biochemical metabolic complexes. Hormones are important modulators. Genes are functionally de-localized and structurally entangled. Genes are plastic and dynamic. Evolutionary biologist Richard Dawkins coined the term "gene cartel" to describe their group significance, and the 1963 Nobel Prize–winner in medicine, Barbara McClintock, discovered the phenomenon of gene flux, or gene mobility. Genes are often redundant, so that the notion of one gene = one function is simply not valid, though it remains a widely accepted paradigm in the public imagination.

We know that thousands of genes are involved in the construction of an eye, a heart, a brain, etc. In the case of diseases, a recent estimate suggests that only about 2 percent of known diseases are triggered by a single gene. Far more commonly, complexity reigns. It is said that even an identified genetic disease such as cystic fibrosis has 350 different gene profiles in its description. A helpful suggestion is to think of the gene not as an independent agent but as one that plays a participating role in complex, dynamic processes. Those processes typically involve the creation of proteins that cause the transformation of energy into structure, new cells that become building blocks of various functional ensembles.

An approach widely used to determine how much of any particular process is due to genetic contributions is to investigate the health history of identical twins. If genes were the only determining factor, and the other three agencies were only negligible factors in assuring health, identical twins would die more or less simultaneously of the same disease. The actual situation is far from the case. Common neurological diseases (Parkinson's and Alzheimer's diseases, especially) of older persons have been shown to have little or no concordance among twins.

Further studies of identical and fraternal twins indicate that heredity accounts for as little as 15 to 20 percent of the differences in human longevity. A study of Swedish twins published in 1998 seems to establish an upper limit of the genetic contribution to 33 percent. It is now generally assumed that the genetic contributions to our overall health and our prospects for longevity fall within a range around 20 percent to 25 percent.

EXTERNAL FACTORS:
INFECTIOUS DISEASE AND ACCIDENTS

Throughout history, the major threat to human health has been an adverse encounter with an external threat. That threat could range from an attack by a predator, an assault by a bullet or a spear, or the intrusion of a virus. Consequences range from the trivial to the fatal.

Medical science has earned the greater part of its acclaim by finding ways of dealing with external agencies—injuries, infections, and infectious diseases. It is these factors that have shaped the medical institutions we know today.

The issue of prevention is important when considering external agency as a health determinant. Most cases of infection, injury, and malignancy are preventable; moreover, it is a lot easier, and obviously cheaper, to prevent them rather than cure them. Or as nineteenth-century American physician and poet Oliver Wendell Holmes wrote, "The shield is nobler than the spear."

INTERNAL FACTORS: MAINTENANCE

Our original car metaphor is nowhere more relevant than in internal agency, the maintenance factor. It is easy enough to imagine the consequences of a poorly maintained car in general. Well-maintained cars can look and perform as new indefinitely. Poorly maintained ones show their age prematurely and have shorter life spans.

Imagine running a car on an inferior grade of gas, or gas that has been contaminated or compromised in some way, for a long period of time. Or using improper motor oil, or never changing the oil at all. Or failing to keep the tires inflated. These (and many other) examples of poor maintenance result in systemic failures of the car in ways that are widely familiar—and prolonged maintenance failure results in a process of cascading failures where a breakdown in one part will lead to a breakdown in another and then another, and so on until the car simply can't run anymore.

The human body's internal agency has two principal components, nutrition and exercise. Both are legacies of our evolutionary past and the crux of our lifestyle choices. The fact that our bodies are extraordinarily complex compounds the problem. Increasing complexity in any system always means increasing opportunities for things to go awry.

Early man, as has been noted, suffered an abbreviated life span primarily as a result of starvation or predation, like most animals. The need to hedge against starvation has given us an affinity for calorically dense foods (which, by the way, are not found in nature but are a product of modern food processing technology). In a mere instant on the human timeline, both our threats and our habits have been radically transformed. As a result, we are witnessing an epidemic of obesity and its consequences, particularly type 2 diabetes. Even more of a revelation is the finding of a recent World Health Organization (WHO) study, claiming that for the first time in human history, the planet has more overweight than underweight people.

A generation ago, severely overweight children were relatively rare.

Now they are commonplace, and in many places the norm. Largely because of this obesity surge, the Centers for Disease Control has noted that the current generation of children may be the first generation since our country was founded that will have a shorter life expectancy than their parents.

Internal agency is driven by energetics, or the quality of energy flow at the cellular level. In the case of obesity and its correlates, excessive energetic input is the disruptive factor.

Too little energetic input is the result of inactivity. Too much energetic interfacing is known by the term "stress," and too little is known as "disuse." Both have far-reaching negative consequences on the afflicted organism, and both are inadequately recognized as basic health threats. Part of the reason for their lack of recognition is the long timeline from cause to effect. The effects of both disuse and stress make themselves known over a relatively long period of time. Both accumulate by degrees and are not always noticeable as they are happening, which is part of their insidiousness. Stress is meant here in the broadest sense. It includes the mental, psychological stresses so intrinsic to modern life, and those diverse physiological responses elaborated by Canadian endocrinologist Hans Selye, who made the term "stress" such an iconic watchword of our times.

In the simplest terms, then, internal agency is physical fitness, derived from exercise and nutrition and fortified by psychological health.

Much of our current thinking on physical fitness comes from a landmark study directed by Dr. Steven Blair, director of research at the Cooper Clinic in Dallas. Blair's paper, "Physical Fitness and All Causes of Mortality: A Prospective Study of Healthy Men and Women," remains a benchmark in our understanding of the relationship between fitness, health, and mortality. Blair's study tracked 13,344 participants over an eight-year period. Bottom line—the least fit group experienced a three- to fourfold greater rate of mortality than the most fit group. There was an unambiguous correlation between fitness and longevity.

> *Blair's group updated their study in a report in 2007. In this case they evaluated 2,603 people over 60 years old for a period of 12 years. The unequivocal health and longevity benefits of fitness pointed to by the first study were verified in this one. The over-60 demographic underscores the message that, instead of "you are too old to exercise," the admonition should be, "you are too old not to exercise."*

Blair's group updated their study in a report in 2007. In this case they evaluated 2,603 people over 60 years old for a period of 12 years. The unequivocal health and longevity benefits of fitness pointed to by the first study were verified in this one. The over-60 demographic underscores the message that, instead of "you are too old to exercise," the admonition should be, "you are too old *not* to exercise."

The benefit is not necessarily from exercise as commonly conceived in the context of a gym or competitive sport activity, but rather the energetics supplied to our cell's receptor sites in a physically active lifestyle that exert strong system-wide effects on all the body's organs and functions that sustain our life processes.

THE AGING PROCESS
AS A HEALTH DETERMINANT

Aging, like life itself, is more than atoms and molecules. It is more than physics and chemistry and is now being seen in terms of the principle of *emergence,* as is the phenomenon of life itself. Emergence can be thought of as the result of numerous simple processes cohering into more complex behaviors when acting in concert, with entirely new properties emerging.

Sixty years ago, French surgeon and biologist Alex Carrell won a Nobel Prize for his demonstration that cells grown in isolation were immortal. This would presume that aging does not apply at the cellular level. Unfortunately, he was wrong. Leonard Hayflick showed conclusively that cells carefully nurtured in cell culture plates have a finite life span. The intracellular details of this programmed aging have yet to be fully worked out, but we know enough to understand that we cannot separate aging from living.

Strictly speaking, aging cannot be reversed. This is not to say, however, that the functions of older individuals are inevitably progressively worse. Stunning improvements that appear to turn back the clock in older people can happen when people utilize previously unrealized phenotypic potential (i.e., our ability to change our physical condition through specific actions such as exercise), a concept that will be explored in detail in subsequent chapters. Importantly, age is never a barrier to phenotypic improvement, leading to one of our favorite maxims about exercise: "It's never too late to start, but it's always too soon to stop."

Using oxygen processing capacity (referred to as oxygen uptake) as an important and instructive example, true age change predicts that the average person will experience a one-half percent per year decline in the ability to process oxygen as fuel. However, if insufficient energy is supplied as a result of inactivity, this rate of decline can be 2 percent or more per year. More importantly, these values can be radically improved with an exercise program for older, unfit people.

Dr. Herbert DeVries's work at the University of Southern California gives some idea of how resiliently we can respond to remedial exercise (that resilience will later be referred to as phenotypic plasticity). DeVries's study group, with an average age of 71, had their oxygen uptakes measured, and then the group submitted to his program of exercise and nutrition. By the end of the study period, the average oxygen uptake measure was equivalent to that of a 28-year-old. This astonishing 40-plus-year differential stands as a profound testimonial to the amount of control we have over the effects of aging.

Studies on patients in nursing homes reveal the real-life benefits from urging residents to retain their vigor and maintain their environ-ments. The fit residents live longer and have fewer hospital visits than their unfit counterparts. Even fit older patients who end up in the ICU do as well as younger patients undergoing similar critical care.

Effectively, we can define aging as "wear and tear, minus repair," or the net difference between the breakdown of our components and our body's effectiveness at rebuild-ing those elements. Our previous studies have shown that the natural rate of aging is approximately one-half of one percent per year. How-ever, when the health of any organ is compromised and its function is impaired, the decline is measurably faster. This is a critical metric of aging, and points up specifically how lifestyle choices are directly correlated with variances from our allotted

DeVries's study group, with an average age of 71, had their oxygen uptakes measured, and then the group submitted to his program of exercise and nutrition. By the end of the study period, the average oxygen uptake measure was equivalent to that of a 28-year-old. This astonishing 40-plus-year differential stands as a profound testimonial to the amount of control we have over the effects of aging.

100 years. Smoking, to cite one obvious example, compromises respiratory function, and lung cells effectively "age" more quickly. Alcoholism can impair liver function and accelerate its decline. And so on.

DIFFERENTIAL AGING

The human body is not a homogeneous mass but rather a networked collection of very different structures and systems. Aging affects different tissues at different rates, and different parts of the body age at different stages. A recent article in New Scientist tells the story of the 80-year-old Norwegian who received a transplant of a 70-year-old cornea 50 years ago. The piece of cornea tissue is now more than 120 years old, and still working, a remarkable example of cellular endurance.

Other organs are made up of very different tissue types. They function in different biochemical and biomechanical environments, with different inputs and outputs. Their missions are radically different. And hence, they tend to age, or lose functional capacity, at differing rates.

Other species have been known to live much longer than humans, which suggests the range of dynamics among living organisms but also gives credence to the notion that longevity is a complex, systemic process that cannot be isolated to a single factor. Among the notable Methuselahs on the planet:

Hexactinellid sponge: 15,000 years

Great Basin bristlecone pine: 4,731 years

Epibenthic sponge: 1,550 years

Ocean quahog: 400 years

Bowhead whale: 211 years

Rougheye rockfish: 205 years

Red sea urchin: 200 years

Many studies have been conducted on long-lived populations in specific geographic locations. Recently the *National Geographic* focused on abnormally high centenarian populations in Okinawa, Japan; Sardinia, Italy; and Loma Linda, California (this last was a concentration of Seventh-Day Adventists). All of these cases revealed that lifestyles, rather than any genetic factors, were the key underlying cause of longevity.

CHAPTER 2

THE EQUIVALENCE OF
DISUSE AND AGING

THE MOTION IMPERATIVE

Life begins with motion. Motion is a metaphor for health and for life itself. It is also what we were designed for. We were born to move. The opposite of motion is stillness—a metaphor for death.

Movement is much more than just walking and running, though. All of life moves, even its most primitive forms. Bacteria move, and not just in some random passive way but in a purposeful manner that assures the two basic elements of life, metabolism and reproduction.

As one ascends the evolutionary ladder, it is increasingly apparent that any animal, when incapacitated by injury, starvation, heat, cold, or age, is at increased risk of death. Paleolithic tribes were forced to abandon members who could no longer walk. Crippled animals in the wild have no recourse and perish. Movement is not simply an indication of life; it is essential to live.

An associated corollary story about the importance of movement to brain development concerns the sea squirt. This primitive sea creature starts out life as a motile larva, eating whatever it can catch. Its movements are under the control of its cerebral ganglion, a simple form of brain. Then it attaches itself to a coral head and abandons its free-living lifestyle, eating only food that happens to drift by. As the sea squirt becomes less dependent on its movement capacity, it needs its brain less and less, and it eventually extrudes its brain and eats it!

Up and down the species ladder we see that animals that move more have bigger brains. Moreover, species that become domesticated tend to have smaller brains as a result of domestication and the attendant constraints it puts on their mobility. For humans, there is a strong suggestion that the reason that our "sapient" brain grew so enormously—three times bigger than our chimpanzee first cousins'—is that we became "persistence hunters" with the attendant higher energy expenditure that that entails, and thereby required a bigger cerebral cortex. Recent neurochemistry research reveals that exercise is a potent stimulus for the critical substance, brain-derived neurotrophic factor (BDNF), which is central to brain development and growth.

Our bodies contain an astonishing 600-plus skeletal muscles that articulate our movements. We have 230 movable or slightly movable joints, and if there are six degrees of freedom (ability to move in either direction along three different axes) for each of them, that means we have 1,380 basic movements that are under our muscular control. Now consider this: Watching people move from a distance, it is often fairly easy to categorize them as "young" or "old" without being close enough to see their features, because of the way they move. The movements of older people tend to be noticeably less fluid and constrained within a smaller range of motion. They exhibit obvious signs of regressive loss of those ranges of motion.

Our ability to move in all the ways we were designed to is a metric of successful aging because it is a primary indicator of our ability to function. What we know from an abundance of studies is that regular use of all our capabilities is the only way of ensuring that our abilities can be sustained. Limited use will inhibit a joint's energetic responses to replenish connective tissue and to produce synovial fluid that lubricates the joint and serves as a shock absorber as well as nourishes the surrounding cartilage. The consequences are the chronic woes of joint pain and inflammation that immobilize so many in their later years.

DISUSE AND AGING

Anyone who suffers a broken leg and the indignity of having that leg immobilized in a cast for several months experiences the shock of seeing a radically altered limb when the cast is removed. In most cases, the affected leg looks like an "old" leg. It appears withered, with a loss of muscle volume and tone. Even its color is pallid. It looks like it has aged a great deal. All of this merely from lack of use.

There is a good reason for this, and it's embedded in our evolutionary heritage. Our genetic makeup is shaped to support the balance between energy intake and energy expenditure that was common to hunter-gatherer societies. Aside from a handful of rather minor genetic adaptations that have occurred since the agricultural revolution, such as lactase tolerance in Caucasians, we are genetically identical to our stone-age precursors.

Paleolithic man lived by moving and usually by running. A variety of forensic approaches have estimated that the typical stone-age adult consumed five times the energy of his modern equivalent. Analyses of fossil bone structure give clues about the size, weight, and kinds of activities that made up our ancestors' daily lives. It is generally believed that they would spend a day or more at a time moving quickly, often at a run, in pursuit of game. When the hunt was successful, they then had to carry the game back to camp, which may have been even more energetically challenging than the original pursuit. We are invited to imagine our ancestors doing a daily cross-country run of 10 miles or so, and then lugging a 50-pound animal all the way back.

Paleolithic women had a roughly equivalent energetic profile. Waking hours were consumed with work, including much of the "gathering" as well as most of the food preparation, the making of clothing and shelter, the transport of camps, and some hunting as well. The differences in caloric expenditure between men and women were not significant.

The agricultural revolution brought about the first major change in that routine. The caloric expenditure associated with raising crops is significant by modern standards, to be sure, but vastly less than that associated with the hunter-gatherer lifestyle. The industrial revolution of the nineteenth century witnessed another quantum decline in energetic requirements as we created tools and engines to take over many of the tasks that had until then been subordinated to muscle power. And finally we are now witnessing the fruits of the digital revolution: Societies are even more indolent, and we tend to see exercise as a luxury that one acquires through memberships in pricey gyms and health clubs.

It is no coincidence that this latter "revolution" is correlated with a horrendous rise in worldwide obesity and type 2 diabetes, as well as a national health care crisis of catastrophic proportions. Various national surveys indicate that as many as four out of every ten adults in the United States are largely inactive. That is, they have sedentary jobs, engage in no particular physical activity or recreation, and are generally inactive around the house.

Dr. Steven Blair of the University of South Carolina's Arnold School of Public Health was senior editor of the 1996 Surgeon General's Report on Physical Activity and Health, and is a professor of exercise science and epidemiology. A large-scale longitudinal study under the direction of Dr. Blair has tracked more than 80,000 adults since 1970. Study participants have been regularly tested, measured, and interviewed; study staff have been tracking their medical histories, body composition, and body mass index, and assessing their stress levels and other lifestyle factors. From these data, Dr. Blair has concluded bluntly that sedentary lives can be deadly, and in fact are a leading cause of early mortality.

The study indicates that fitness level is a significant predictor of mortality. One major follow-up study of more than 40,000 participants determined that poor fitness levels accounted for 16 percent of all deaths, regardless of gender. This figure was derived from estimates of the number of deaths that would have been avoided if the subjects had simply had a nominal measure of fitness. Just 30 minutes a day of walking would add six years to the life span of an inactive person.

Further examination of nearly 15,000 women in the program showed that women who were very fit were also 55 percent less likely to die of breast cancer than women who were notably unfit. This remarkable fact was revealed after other known risk factors—including body mass index (BMI), smoking, and family history of breast cancer—and other known risk factors had been accounted for.

These findings were unflinchingly presented at the annual convention of the American Psychological Association under the title "Physical Inactivity: The Biggest Public Health Problem of the 21st Century." Blair notes that, over the past few decades, we have largely engineered the need for physical activity out of the daily lives of most people in contemporary society, and adds that the message is simple—doing *something* is better than doing nothing; doing *more* is better than doing less (up to a reasonable point). Our own inactivity is the greatest challenge facing our public health agenda.

Another longitudinal study, this time by a team of Harvard researchers, followed a group of 2,357 men with a mean age of 72 who were generally in good health. The study sought data on the non-genetic determinants of exceptional longevity. The study sought conclusive evidence associated with modifiable factors, that is, lifestyle choices associated with a life span of 90 years or greater. They found that regular exercise resulted in a nearly 30 percent lower mortality risk, and that those with healthy lifestyle choices (those who got regular exercise, were non-smokers, and had no hypertension, diabetes, or obesity) at the age of 70 had a 54 percent chance of living to 90 or beyond. In addition, those healthy participants reported better late-life physical function and mental well-being, as well as a lower incidence of the chronic diseases usually associated with aging. Regular exercise stood out as the key determinant of healthy, functional longevity.

USE IT OR LOSE IT

It is abundantly clear that inactivity negatively impacts good health and, in fact, foreshortens one's potential life span. In the analytic repertoire of contemporary clinical medicine, there has been no coherent way of classifying the effects that we now see as a result of inactivity. The standard medical model, which seeks external agents (viruses and other pathogens) as the cause of diseases, has hampered a full understanding of aging physiology. In fact, we now know that many diseases that are so prevalent in older persons are distinct and separable from the process of aging itself. They arise instead from extended periods of inactivity.

Inactivity can actually be deadly. Going to bed for 72 hours lowers glucose utilization by 50 percent. The incidence of diabetes is substantially increased after spinal cord injury or any injury that hinders mobility.

We can classify this phenomenon as Disuse Syndrome. It includes a broad spectrum of diseases or degenerative declines that are generally associated with older people. These include:

- *Muscle and bone weakness.* Muscle tissue will lose mass and tone without stimulation. Bones require the energetics of circulation and stress to maintain their structural integrity and living processes.

Osteoporosis and muscular weakness are not inevitable by-products of aging.

- *Immune system compromise.* Moderate exercise causes immune cells to circulate more rapidly and do a more effective job of attacking viruses and bacteria. When exercise ends, the immune response returns to normal in a matter of hours. Regular exercise, however, extends the benefit even longer. Studies by Professor David Nieman of Appalachian State University revealed that a regular program of moderate exercise creates a cumulative effect that reinforces long-term immune response. For instance, subjects in the study who walked at 70–75 percent of their maximum heart rate for 40 minutes per day reported only half as many sick days as those who didn't exercise.

- *Narrowing of the arteries* (atherosclerosis). Our arteries are our lifelines, literally, carrying blood from our heart to keep our vital organs and life processes nourished and functional. Atherosclerosis is the leading cause of death and disability in the industrialized world today, via heart attacks and strokes. Arterial narrowing is connected to a broad spectrum of other issues as well, such as glaucoma. A study by Greek scientists found that aerobic exercise, including vigorous exercise, unequivocally benefited glaucoma patients by reducing inter-ocular pressure.

- *Metabolic decline.* Our metabolic rate is a measure of how well our "engine" is running. A declining metabolic resting rate has generally been considered an expected consequence of aging. But a number of recent studies have successfully challenged that assumption with the hypothesis that age-related decline in resting metabolic rate is not observed in people who exercise regularly. One study, of a group of women that included both sedentary postmenopausal subjects and postmenopausal distance runners and swimmers, showed striking results. The group of endurance athletes showed not only faster (that is, more youthful) metabolic rates but also a notable resistance to body fat and weight gain.

- *Central nervous system compromise.* We are on the threshold of understanding the link between physical fitness and central nervous system health in a quantifiable way. A number of recent studies all point to a correlation between an active lifestyle and the absence of degenerative diseases associated with aging, including Alzheimer's and Parkinson's. It is no coincidence that, virtually without exception, physically healthy centenarians are remarkably free of these debilitating conditions. Adding to this, a new study claims that obesity, disuse's partner in crime, is associated with "severe brain degeneration," which is associated with loss of brain tissue and resultant premature aging of the brain. Cells die and fail to be fully replaced because of a lack of energetic stimuli.

- *Frailty.* Frailty, a term that sums up all the adverse effects of aging, has only recently achieved recognition as a syndrome in its own right, largely due to extensive research at Johns Hopkins University. Frailty affects the entire body, particularly the muscles, the skeleton, and the neural and endocrine systems. It is widely prevalent in older adults and is typically the culprit in the all-too-familiar falls and fractures that the elderly endure. Frailty is particularly pernicious because it means loss of function, which means loss of independent capabilities. We can define frailty as a state of 30 percent or less of original functional capability.

  Leg strength appears to be a key indicator of frailty. Dr. Jack Guralnik of the National Institutes of Health's National Institute on Aging has shown that leg power, not age or disease state, is the single best predictor of a subsequent need for nursing home placement. The legs may well be the most important physical element in the aging person's body, more so than heart, lungs, and brain, because healthy legs can improve the health of all the other organs. Legs are our principal source of motive power, our greatest source of energy production by far. The vast majority of aerobic exercise comes from movement driven by leg power.

Each of these factors is the explicit by-product of consistent, long-term disuse. They are related in terms of energy throughput, or more accurately, a deficit of energy production and exchange at the receptor sites of specific groups of cells. Without a consistent flow of energy at the cellular level, the efficiency of our basic internal processes begins to degrade. This formulation of the Disuse Syndrome was anticipated by earlier designations of the rise of activity-related health issues, beginning with the label "hypokinetic disease" in the early 1960s. The term Sedentary Death Syndrome, or SeDS, was coined in an initial attempt to bring attention to the more than 300,000 deaths per year in the United States that can be attributed to long-term disuse.

We are awash in data from every part of the globe that confirm how dangerous disuse is. While the populace of the United States may be indisputably the worst offenders, the syndrome now has global reach. For instance, a long-term Swedish study analyzing the energy expenditures of 33,000 men concluded that modern life has resulted in an energetic drop-off for the average citizen equivalent to 45 minutes of brisk daily walking.

A noted experiment in Australia had seven men go off into the bush and live like original settlers from 150 years ago. Over a period of a week, the subjects were found to have used 2.3 times more energy each day than in their normal lives, which turned out to be the equivalent of walking an additional ten miles each day. In England, it was determined that between 1945 and 1995, the average adult caloric expenditure declined by 800 calories per day. Again, this worked out to the equivalent of a ten-mile-per-day walk. Interestingly, present-day hunter-gatherers, like the bushmen of the Kalahari, have been estimated to move 11.5 miles per day on average.

In Hong Kong, a study carried out by the University of Hong Kong and the Department of Health looked at the level of physical activity in people who had died, and were able to correlate their level of physical activity with their risk of dying. The results indicated that 20 percent of all deaths of people 35 and older could be attributed to a lack of physical activity. That is greater than the number of deaths associated with smoking. The study also showed that the risk of dying from cancer increased 45 percent for men and 28 percent for women as a consequence of inactivity. The risk of dying from respiratory ailments was 92 percent higher for men and 75 percent higher for women. The risk of dying from heart disease was 52 percent higher for men and 28 percent higher for women, all due to a lack of physical activity.

> *Again, this worked out to the equivalent of a ten-mile-per-day walk. Interestingly, present-day hunter-gatherers, like the bushmen of the Kalahari, have been estimated to move 11.5 miles per day on average.*

Worldwide, physical inactivity now rates as one of the major health issues in the modern world. It is estimated to be the primary cause of 1.9 million premature deaths annually. Globally, physical inactivity is identified as a causal factor in 10 to 16 percent of breast cancers, colon cancers, and diabetes, and about 22 percent of ischemic heart disease.

There is a glut of shocking statistics to support the negative effects of disuse, from every angle of modern life. There is not a single demonstrable fact or statistic making a case for the desirability of inactive lifestyles. But after a while information that should be a clarion call to personal and political action merely makes us numb. There is too much, and it is too overwhelming.

> *Globally, physical inactivity is identified as a causal factor in 10 to 16 percent of breast cancers, colon cancers, and diabetes, and about 22 percent of ischemic heart disease.*

All of the laborsaving devices and gadgets of contemporary life come with a caloric price tag. The table on page 49 illustrates one study's computation of the differences between caloric output associated with a variety of ordinary daily activities.

The cumulative impact of machines was estimated at 111 calories per day, or the equivalent of 45 minutes of walking.

A partial list of diseases or conditions that can be caused or exacerbated by chronic inactivity includes:

Aneurysm

Angina

Atherosclerosis

Back pain

Cardiovascular diseases

Colorectal cancer

Coronary heart disease

Diabetes

Hemorrhoids

Hypertension

Kidney stones

Osteoarthritis

Osteoporosis

Type 2 diabetes

The central role that physical activity plays in regulating total body energy balance and therefore the odds of getting or not getting obese or diabetic cannot be over-emphasized, particularly in light of the epidemic of inactivity noted above. We are moving less and less, and "use it or lose it" has never been a more powerful or compelling admonition.

Table 2.1

Activity	Caloric Output, Manual	Caloric Output, Machine
Washing dishes	45	27
Doing laundry	80	54
Going upstairs	11 (stairs)	3 (escalator)
Getting to work	83 (walking)	25 (driving)

MOLECULAR AGE VERSUS
CHRONOLOGICAL AGE

King's College, London, maintains the largest database of twins in the world, for a variety of studies. Twin studies are particularly useful in research because observed differences between pairs of twins can point conclusively to causes that might otherwise be confounding or difficult to sort out. Having common DNA portrayed against significant differences can unequivocally indicate non-genetic causes.

A research team at King's College sought evidence of aging at a molecular level by investigating telomeres in a large study group of twins. Telomeres, as pointed out in the previous chapter, serve as protective "caps" at the end of our chromosomes to help prevent them from damage. As we age, our telomeres shorten with each cell division, leaving our cells more vulnerable to disease.

The study population was comprised of both identical twins and fraternal twins. Comparing the telomere lengths of twins who were raised together but who experienced different amounts of exercise showcases the effect of environmental variation within a common gene set, and so provides a more powerful test of the Disuse Syndrome hypothesis. On average, the telomeres of the more active twin were significantly longer than those of the less active twin. The effect of activity

as a cause of increased longevity clearly overshadowed the genetic contribution. Nurture trumped nature.

The study found an even more alarming result: A sedentary lifestyle
may diminish life expectancy not only by predisposing someone to age-
related diseases but by hastening the aging process itself. The investigators found that telomere length decreased steadily with age, as
expected. But there was a significant association between increasing
physical activity and longer telomere length even after adjusting for
other measurable influences,
particularly body weight, smoking, and socioeconomic status.
This means the converse is also
true: that inactivity or disuse provides the quickest route to
telomere shortening. In this case,

*At the University of North Carolina,
a major research project has been
seeking ways to determine our actual
"molecular" age in contrast to our
chronological age.*

the correlation between level of activity and telomere shortening was
dramatic. The difference in telomere length between the most active
subjects and the inactive subjects corresponds to around *nine years of aging*.

At the University of North Carolina, it was found in a study reported
in the journal *Aging Cell* that as tissue ages, concentrations of a certain
protein (called p16INK4a in the code used by microbiologists) dramatically increase. The protein is present in the T-cells of the immune

system, which play a key role in fighting disease and repairing tissue damage. Researchers discovered that not only is the protein a biological
marker for cellular aging, but its presence is also directly correlated with
physical inactivity. In the quest to find a simple blood test to detect the
protein levels, test subjects were extensively queried, revealing that level
of physical activity appears to be the most significant of all lifestyle factors as a means of slowing down cellular aging, outstripping all other factors, including obesity and smoking.

A study at the University of California, Berkeley, sought to identify
the critical biochemical pathways linked to the aging of human muscle
tissue. Previous research in animal models revealed that the ability of
adult stem cells to repair and replace damaged tissue is governed by the
molecular signals they get from surrounding muscle tissue, and that
those signals tend to change with age in ways that inhibit tissue repair.
Those studies have also shown that regenerative old stem cells can be re-
vived with the appropriate biochemical signals. What was not clear until
this new study was whether similar rules applied for humans. Unlike
humans, laboratory animals are bred to have identical genes and are
raised in similar environments. Moreover, the typical human life span
lasts seven to eight decades, while lab mice are reaching the end of their
lives after two years.

In experiments conducted on two groups of subjects, one consist-
ing of men in their early twenties and the other in their late sixties and
early seventies, muscle biopsies were taken from the quadriceps of all the

subjects at the beginning of the study. The men then had the leg from which the muscle tissue was taken immobilized in a cast for two weeks to simulate muscle atrophy. After the cast was removed, the study participants exercised with weights to regain muscle mass in their newly freed legs. Analysis of the muscle tissue showed that older muscles, having had a much longer period of disuse, responded much more slowly. The study inferred that very long periods of disuse can degrade the cells' regenerative environment. Hence the conclusion that regeneration of human muscle tissue in "old" muscles is markedly enhanced by continuous attention to fitness. "Use it or lose it" is an imperative, right down to the cellular level.

Numerous large observational studies address the inactivity/obesity/diabetes/mortality axes. An eight-year review of 70,000 nurses revealed over 1,400 new cases of diabetes. The less fit nurses had double the incidence of diabetes of the more fit. A Physicians Health Study of more than 20,000 doctors revealed a five-year incidence of new diabetes, again with a 50 percent protection factor by fitness. A Cooper Aerobic Center study showed that unfit men were four times as likely to become diabetic than fit men. An extensive survey of 35,000 women in Minnesota revealed that *any* amount of physical activity lowered the incidence of new diabetes by 30 percent. Another, in Malmö, Sweden, reviewed the life history of a group of people who showed early signs of diabetes—such as high blood sugar levels—and found that an exercise intervention lowered their mortality rate to that of persons who were not pre-diabetic. Exercise effectively "cured" prediabetes at least as far as mortality was concerned. That is, those who used exercise as an intervention did not die as a result of eventual diabetes.

Geneticist Mae-Wan Ho, director of the Institute of Science in Society, summarizes the destructive consequences of inactivity in no uncertain terms:

> Inactivity starves our tissues and cells of oxygen and hence energy for metabolic activities. It also leads to a build-up of reactive oxygen species that cause oxidative damages to the cells including DNA, that would further inhibit anabolic (constructive) activities, if not encourage downright catabolic (destructive) tendencies. In the wider context, inactivity leads to a loss of (quantum) coherence and balance in the "energy field," which I certainly would not dismiss.

Inactivity, or disuse, is clearly a scourge of our time and our culture, and the single leading cause of health issues. The correlation between physical activity and extended life spans is compelling. "Physical activity" is an enormously broad term, and while any sensible activity is surely beneficial, we need to look deeper into the internal mechanisms that keep us alive and well to understand the full arc of the longest and healthiest possible life.

CHAPTER 3

FOUNDATIONS OF
SUCCESSFUL AGING

A TIP FROM THE ORACLE

Humans are masterworks of evolution, the most successfully adaptive of all life forms. Yet it's likely that only a few of us fully understand—or fully appreciate—just how remarkable we are.

If there were a first rule of longevity, it would be the command "*Know thyself*," handed down to us from the Delphic Oracle some 3,000 years ago. Our bodies constantly give us feedback on our internal workings. Our central nervous system is an ingeniously complex network that provides us with a wide array of information about our well-being and the threats to it. So much that it's a challenge for most of us to monitor and process.

Competitive athletes tend to be acutely aware of changes in their bodies. They will raise an alarm over small variations of which the majority of us might be entirely unaware. Most of the rest of us, however, learn to tune out all but the most acute of the signals. We take what happens inside us for granted, oblivious to everything but our internal signals with the general exceptions of fatigue, acute pain, and hunger. But pain and discomfort occur on many levels and gradations. To the extent that we are aware of them, our recognition threshold is rather high. Early warning signs slip by unnoticed, and we don't realize that things aren't right until they are considerably out of whack.

Our bodies are wonderfully complex machines, made up of something on the order of hundreds of trillions of cells, each of which interacts with other individual cells as well as in functional aggregates. And yet we manage to experience homeostasis, or the ability of an organism to maintain its equilibrium by adjusting its internal processes. Our ability to maintain a constant temperature of 98.6 degrees is a simple example of homeostasis.

We compared the human body to a car in Chapter 1 in order to make a key point about maintenance. To take the analogy further, if we have a cheap clunker, we are likely not to pay much attention to unsettling sounds coming from a poorly maintained engine, a slipping transmission, the rattles of the chassis, and the loosened fittings. But should we find ourselves in possession of an expensive high-performance sports car, we would likely be acutely aware of every note in its mechanical orchestra, every minute deviation from its perfect natural harmonics.

We all have that choice with respect to our *corpus,* our physical condition. Will we be the "clunker" that we pray will get us down the road each day, or the high-performance machine that may require meticulous maintenance but will carry us much farther and provide the highest levels of enjoyment and satisfaction?

THE PROCESSES OF LIFE

That high-performance sports car that we covet as a model for our physical functioning has components that work perfectly in concert. The clunker that we cite as the antithesis is likely out of tune, its ignition and exhaust mismatched, its wheels out of balance, its tires out of alignment. Each degradation of a component induces compromises in other parts of the system. And so it is with our bodies, though we are vastly more complex, more intricate. But the analogy underscores the necessity of knowing ourselves as systems, not just a collection of functions such as respiration, digestion, circulation, and so on.

We used the term "homeostasis" above in the context of our ability to maintain the basic equilibrium necessary to support our internal workings in a safe, stable way. "Stasis" is the limiting term here, indicating processes that work toward a static or fixed objective. Our internal environment is a foundation of homeostatic processes that regulate temperature, acidity, ionic composition, and an array of other biochemical metrics.

But of course, we change. We age. We decay. Or maybe we embark on a fitness program and build ourselves up and increase our physical capabilities. These changes are the result of system-wide processes that we will refer to as homeodynamics—that is, processes that dynamically direct the overall changes in our bodies in response to specific energetic inputs that we bring to bear on ourselves.

Our lifelines are not purely homeostatic: They begin at conception, and end at death. We are born, develop, mature, and age. Our homeostatic mechanisms are not themselves constant during the arc of our lives, but change over time. As organisms, we are active players in our own fate, not simply the unwitting victims of nature, the gods, or even natural selection. To understand our lifelines, therefore, we need to tune into what our bodies are telling us; we need to think beyond homeostasis and focus on the much more robust and richer concept of homeodynamics. Whereas homeostasis is part of what defines us as a species, homeodynamics is what makes each of us unique as our bodies maintain biochemical individuality by constantly undergoing physiologic and metabolic processes. Homeodynamics is the constantly changing interrelatedness of body components while an overall equilibrium is maintained.

A simple example of homeodynamics can be seen as a consequence of the way our maximal heart rate decreases linearly with age, one of the natural consequences of aging. But because we require the same basic amount of blood flow to service our body, our heart increases the amount of blood it pumps with each stroke, compensating for the decline in maximum rate.

In concert with homeodynamics, another unwieldy term rises to help us understand our metabolic processes and their relation to our lifelines, *symmorphosis.* Symmorphosis is the process by which we undergo specific changes as a result of the energetic environment we provide for ourselves. It is the unifying concept underlying our physiology, operating much like a master engineering protocol that determines how all our components will work in parallel. Beyond the foundation concept of "form follows function" is the more general rule, form follows function, *subject to the boundaries of the total energetic environment.* The gene ensembles, through homeodynamic processes, obey deterministic energetic principles. The whole organism performs best when the metabolism and genes are integrated and harmonic. This, then, is health, the emergent state of the entire organism, when all the components are optimally tuned to their specified functions, when all systems are working as they are supposed to.

This leads us to the central concept of phenotypic plasticity. We speak of genotype and phenotype as the yin and yang of our unique descriptors. Genotype refers to the genetic information with which we come encoded. Phenotype refers to our observed properties, or what we become. Genotype is nature; phenotype is nurture. Strictly speaking, phenotypic plasticity is the production of multiple phenotypes from a single genotype. What it means to us is the effect environment has on the expression of genetic potential.

Plasticity is the most crucial factor in health and longevity. It is the living, physical expression of the lifestyle choices we make. It is the most powerful tool that nature has put at our disposal, the ability to shape ourselves and to control our health and our physical destiny. We have the capability, through actions of our choice, to alter our muscle mass and strength, to improve our oxygen processing capacity, to literally improve the functionality of our cells, including our brain cells.

> *We have the capability, through actions of our choice, to alter our muscle mass and strength, to improve our oxygen processing capacity, to literally improve the functionality of our cells, including our brain cells.*

Phenotypic plasticity has barely made it into our medical lexicon, but it is destined to be an elemental part of our future understanding of living systems. We see it all around us, though we're rarely aware of it. It is most obvious in plants, because they stay fixed in position while they grow and change according to the interplay of their genetics and their environmental inputs. We hike up a mountain and watch the same species of tree, with a common genotype, change in structure and appearance as we go higher and higher, which means we are witnessing the trees under changing conditions of sunlight, growing season, soil type, weather, and competing plant species.

The restorative and regenerative powers of our native plasticity are evolution's most generous and useful bequeathal to us. They have given us a remarkable amount of control over our physical well-being. Unlike plants, which must make a go of it wherever they happen to take root, and have no ability to alter their environment, we have a vast array of choices about lifestyle and environment. Considering how few things in life are within our span of control, it's astonishing that this fact isn't more appreciated. In biology, this is called "niche construction," and it is the embodiment of our ability to shape our physical destiny. Our adaptability, our plasticity, effectively puts less of a burden on our genes to define us. We become what we do.

From homeostasis to homeodynamics, to symmorphosis to phenotypic plasticity. This daunting array of terminology falls under the general rubric of systems biology and the new science of *emergence*. The progress of science—and of health and medicine—has historically been a pattern of reductive analysis. Reductionism seeks to explain complex phenomena in terms of ever smaller components, by digging down progressively deeper and sorting out the minutiae. It has been a remarkably successful intellectual discipline so far, giving us knowledge of the fine-grained structure of the universe as well as the microscopic agents of infectious diseases, among other things.

THE REDUCTIONIST FALLACY—
NO MAGIC BULLETS

But reductionism has led to a dead end in many areas, particularly health. It has burdened us with the expectation of "magic bullets," the notion that illness (and aging) arise from specific isolated sources and are remediable by simplistic measures. We look to technology to provide the "anti-aging" potion, pill, or surgical procedure. In fact, respected scientists have gone on the record for decades predicting just such advances. But no breakthroughs have materialized.

The futurist Ray Kurzweil predicted in *Fantastic Voyage: The Science Behind Radical Life Extension,* a book speculating on possibilities for living indefinitely, that, "before the ink is dry" on the book, at least one of his predictions would have materialized. None did. Five years later, his latest book advises us to hold on another 20 years or so for advances like DNA reprogramming and submicroscopic (nanotechnology) cell-repairing robots. A central problem with all of these proposed life-extension solutions is that they all seem to focus on a single target, whereas aging is a complex, system-wide phenomenon. Hence the imperative for systemic approaches. We may, in fact, be able to employ nanotechnology for certain repairs at the cellular level. And we are already making stunning advances in genetic engineering. But no one has yet slowed down (much less stopped!) the aging process. There is not a centenarian alive today who would ascribe his or her longevity to a drug, a pill, or any form of new technology acquired through the medical establishment.

The likelihood of there ever being an anti-aging pill is in the same ballpark as the infamous metaphorical free lunch. No such thing. Even if medical technology were to find an ingestible substance that inhibited aging, we have no idea what the unintended consequences might be at the cellular level. What other fundamental biochemical processes might be affected? In medicine this goes by the deceptively benign term "side effects."

Gene therapy is an instructive example. In what was regarded as the first successful deployment of gene therapy, a treatment program for sufferers of severe combined immune deficiency (SCID) was launched in 1990. Less than a decade later, some of the subjects began to die. A number succumbed to leukemia, as it was eventually determined that the therapy interfered with a gene that can trigger cancer.

But what, you might ask, about all the promising new treatments popping up with regularity in the popular media? A great deal of money is being invested in creating and marketing products that claim to slow down or stop the shrinkage of telomeres, the "caps" on our DNA strands. But after years of investment, not to mention a barrage of marketing hype, there are still no conclusive studies to support the viability of such a method.

What about the various treatments that are extending the life spans of everything from yeasts to nematodes to laboratory rats? What about the "miracle" substance derived from red wine grapes, resveratrol? Despite widespread acclaim, purveyors all over the Internet, and an appearance on *60 Minutes* by its leading proponent, resveratrol has yet to conclusively show any long-term benefit to humans.

Experiments on yeasts, flatworms, and small mammals are all necessary first steps, to be sure. In fact, longevity treatments are tested on subjects like these precisely because of their very short life spans. Fruit flies, *drosophila,* have a life cycle of about two weeks. A treatment that promised a 50 percent extension of life span could be observed over a mere three-week period. Standard testing on humans is obviously constrained by the long periods of observation required. While it is encouraging to see impressive life extension results in animal subjects, the fact remains that other animals have very different metabolic processes from our own, and we know that we cannot simply assume that the results of those experiments carry over to humans.

There is no commercially available substance, no treatment, no therapy, no procedure available today that can demonstrably extend life or protect us from the various ravages of aging. This is remarkable considering how many products are being promoted with just such promises. It requires no stretch of critical thinking to note that, if any of these were categorically successful, we would know about it in a dramatic way.

Verifiable success stories would be headline news, and the product name would be a household word. It is no coincidence that most of these get-young-quick products come with fine print that informs the user that they work best in conjunction with diet and exercise!

The limitations of reductionism as well as the ongoing failure to come up with singly targeted life extension solutions is leading to an increasing movement toward a systemic or system-wide approach. The growing emphasis on systems biology is an important outgrowth of this movement away from reductionism. The systems approach culminates in the concept of *emergence,* and from this we recognize health as an emergent property. A system expresses new features that could not be detected in any one of the system's elements. By this standard, we can see that illness is a disruption of one or more parts of the system, thereby preventing the expression of one of the system's emergent properties.

We can summarize thus: No part of us is an island—no one cell, no one gene, no one organ, stands alone. Health is a property of our total system, which is a synthesis of all its components and processes. Our genotype contains the boundaries for our potential; but the expression of our phenotype is what gives us the ability to live to our full potential. Our health is a matter of choice, not fate.

Hence the path to 100 healthy years is a matrix of core variables that we can now identify.

RUNNING FOR YOUR LIFE

We seem to generally accept the idea that running is "good for you." It has long been known that running has immediate cardiovascular benefits. But what of the overall role of running as a mediator of comprehensive health? And what measurable effect might a consistent program of running have on longevity?

At the Stanford University Medical Center, beginning in 1984, some 500 older runners were tracked for more than 20 years, and their health and fitness measured against a similar group of non-runners. The mean age of the subjects at the start of the study was 59. In 1984, the conventional wisdom was that vigorous exercise would most likely be harmful to older people, that the weakening effects of aging would make them susceptible to injury and breakdown. At the very least, the thinking went, there would be orthopedic injuries, particularly knees, ankles, and hips.

The researchers hypothesized that consistent exercise with a high energetic throughput (that is, hard workouts) would enhance and extend the quality of life, and help keep the exerciser free of disabilities. At the time, longevity was not an issue; rather, researchers focused on the idea of minimizing the period toward the end of life when people began to lose their self-efficacy. The idea became known as the "compression of morbidity" theory.

Not surprisingly, the runner group lived longer and healthier lives, with significantly fewer common illnesses or disabilities. What wasn't expected was that the runner group was found to be only half as likely to die from major illnesses, including cancer, neurological diseases, and infections, than the non-running group.

At the beginning of the study period, the participants ran, on average, close to four hours per week. Twenty-one years later, the average had dropped to 76 minutes per week, but that is still around 25 minutes every other day, a very reasonable benchmark for most people, but noteworthy considering the mean age of the group was 78.

Toward the end of the study, with participants now in their seventies and eighties, only 15 percent of the runners had died, compared to 34 percent of the non-runners. For those runners who encountered disabilities during the study period, those disabilities set in a full 16 years later, on average, than they did for the non-runners, a truly startling discovery. The lead investigator, emeritus professor of medicine James Fries, noted, "The study has a very pro-exercise message. If you had to pick one thing to make people healthier as they age, it would be aerobic exercise. The health benefits of exercise are greater than we thought."

Interestingly, biomechanical analysis of the human foot at the University of Calgary makes the case that the shape of our toes indicates how successfully we have evolved as natural runners. Shorter, stubby toes, unlike the long prehensile toes of our primate cousins, are vastly better suited for running, especially over extended distances. Most animals that run also have very short toes. Some species, such as cats and dogs, have paws composed almost entirely of palms.

Few other animals are capable of long-distance running, and none can do so under a blazing sun. Wolves, for instance, require cold weather or nightfall for long-distance hunting; otherwise, they overheat. Endurance running may well have set early humans apart from the rest of the animal kingdom.

According to the University of Calgary study, many of our anatomical features seem particularly adapted to running all day on the savannahs. Achilles tendons act as springs to store energy. Our legs have unusually large joints. Our buttock muscles support balance and stabilization. And regions of our brain appear uniquely sensitive to the physical pitching generated by the motion of running. We are probably the world's best long-distance runners among mammals, though on the other hand, we're very poor sprinters, limited by the mechanics of foot and toe structure.

ALL YOU NEED TO KNOW ABOUT RUNNING

Technique? Put one foot after the other. There's not much more to it. We've been running as long as we've been walking upright as hominids. Don't worry about technique.

Gear? Any running shoe will do. Frankly, the differences between various brands are not likely to make a difference to a novice runner. In fact, there are recent studies suggesting that all the running shoe technology is potentially harmful overkill. It is theorized that too much cushioning creates an unnatural relationship between foot and ground, leading to a variety of potential injuries over time.

Getting chapped when the insides of your upper legs rub together while you run? Use a little Vaseline on your legs. If your feet blister easily, a little Vaseline on a foot can help prevent blister-inducing friction.

Cool or cold weather? Layering is the key. Start out with a windbreaker that you can tie off around your waist once you get warm. It's that simple.

Good running is smooth running. Strive to make the least possible noise as your feet hit the ground. Smoothness means that you're minimizing the shock on your feet and knees and are less likely to be hurting afterward. Run lightly.

Don't run on your toes. Run with a rolling motion over the balls of your feet.

Stretching is best done, and most beneficial, after a run, not before. A little light stretching without full extension beforehand is fine, though.

Don't be intimidated by others. The only person you're competing with is yourself.

RUNNING: A FEMALE PERSPECTIVE

By Ruth Anne Bortz

He says "you can't."
She says "watch me."

Thirty-four years ago, when I was 46 years old, I was the prototypical middle-aged wife, mother, and homemaker. I had four children, a formidable husband, a lovely home, and a life script that seemed close to ideal. Travel was part of the fortunate repertoire of our life at that time. Dragging the kids along, we had lived in Germany for one year during a training period, youth-hosteled through the British Isles for one month, and skied several times in Switzerland as a family, but when a doctor friend showed us his slides of a trip to the Himalayas, we confronted an entirely different level of challenge. Were we—was I—up to the rigorous exertions that such a trek would surely demand?

For my husband uncertainty was not an issue. When his father died, he started to run as a grief response, and carried this habit up to running marathons, so a hike in the high mountains was not daunting for him. I was not so sure about myself. True, I had always been an athlete in school, playing basketball and hockey and tennis with my schoolmates. I had even been a finalist in my college golf tournament. But did this translate to being able to climb to 20,000 feet? Not so sure.

But somehow I did, and I was not the laggard of the group. I found the experience exhilarating. When we emerged from this experience I felt I was in the best shape of my life. There was no mountain I couldn't climb, no marathon I couldn't run.

"You can't do that," I was admonished. "Running a marathon is not in your life script. Sweating is not your style. Running shoes are not your fashion."

"Watch."

I was lucky that I had a close neighbor friend, Nicki Weicker, who shared my interest in getting fit. We met at the mailbox in our new running outfits. Our hair was done, our lipstick was neat, our shoes were tied, so off we went. First two miles, then three, then five. "What's the big deal? We can do this."

We entered a 10K race and did okay, finishing with smiles. My husband smiled too, but still wasn't really convinced. Our kids started to notice and cheer their running mom. Within several months I was entered in my first marathon, the Avenue of the Giants Marathon through the redwoods of Northern California. This event in 1978 marked a rebirth for me. I was reborn as a marathon runner. The fact that I left my husband far behind in the pack was not a coincidence. He ran simply to accumulate the health benefits of running. I ran to win. We developed an entirely different lifestyle with different devotions and different friends. I entered several other marathons and did very well for my age group. Meanwhile, our youngest child, Walter, caught the running bug. He had the advantage of being a beautiful, effortless runner and seemed to cover the miles without strain. In 1981, we had developed friends who were involved in the Western States 100-mile trail run from Squaw Valley to Auburn, California, along an old mining trail. It was certified as the world's toughest endurance test. It spoke mightily to our sense of challenge.

Proudly Walter entered, and prevailed. We watched and cheered, and I wondered: "Can I do it?"

"You can't do that."

"Watch."

And so, in 1984, at the age of 54, I entered, easily the most wildly un-likely experience of my sheltered life. At 5 A.M. under the chairlift at Squaw Valley, at the starting line with my nervous family, I faced 100 miles of un-certainty, of uncharted territory. Over snowfields, through 100-degree canyons, across the American River on a rope, into and through a night with flashlights uncertainly showing the way. The dawn slowly came on me, with my husband, who crewed the last 30 miles, alternately cheering and cursing to urge me the last miles to Auburn, still seeming impossibly dis-tant. At a little after 9 A.M. I entered the track at Auburn high school. There ahead was my cheering family, just as they had been at the start 28 hours and 100 miles earlier.

"Yes, I can!"

Two years later, at age 56, I did the race again, this time four hours faster. I have continued to run ever since, winning trophies for women in the over-60 and over-70 categories in the Boston Marathon. And now this running heritage has spilled over to the younger generations. All four of our children, as well as one grandchild, have completed marathons, and an-other grandchild has it on her calendar. My husband and I plan on run-ning Boston again to celebrate our eightieth birthdays shortly. Then what? Why stop there?

RUNNING: A PERSONAL RETROSPECTIVE

By Walter Bortz

Why run?

Why, might we ask, is the term "Born to Run" the title of a hit song and a best-selling book? Because it is our heritage, with roots that date back millions of years. All of our ancestors were runners. Those who didn't run are not our ancestors—their genes didn't survive to be passed down.

Herbert Spencer proclaimed the principle of survival of the fittest. He didn't know that he was affirming the survival of the fittest genes. While we don't have a simple running gene, most of our 20,000-plus gene ensemble has some relationship to running. Running is good for all our genes, and the reverse—not running—is bad for all our genes. If we don't run, those genes become under-expressed, which is another way of saying that their signals do not get properly activated.

And we can't simply go to the drugstore and buy a fine set of the ideal gene array! Not a chance! Fit genes must be earned the old-fashioned way, by work. Fit genes have a cost that is measured in sweat.

Mankind's adoption of the wheel and electricity has confused the relationship between health and the effort required to achieve it. There is no surrogate for effort. This is the *why* of running.

When to run?

Simple question, simple answer: Run when you can. I'm compelled to run first thing in the morning, before the rest of the day starts to change my priorities. "I don't have the time" is not an acceptable reason not to run. Running is imperative for a healthy lifestyle, and any distraction that short-circuits this lacks authority. When to run? Whenever you can. Just do it, as the ad says.

Where to run?

Not a very difficult question to answer. You run wherever you are, in an apartment or in a hailstorm, at the gymnasium or track, in the neighborhood, on the beach, on hilly trails. When our ancestors were peering out from their lair and saw a potential meal to feed their starving brood grazing nearby, they didn't ponder the circumstances. I relish the worst conditions. One January morning in Chicago, I was slated for a five-mile run. It was bitter cold with a piercing wind and a light snowfall. I neglected to note the direction of the wind, which was blowing north along the lake. I had a tailwind on the way north, but on the way back I recognized my new adversary, a brisk bitter headwind. By the time I returned to the hotel, frost hung from my eyebrows, my nostrils were encrusted, I breathed snowflakes. But I had done it and felt amazingly better for it.

The converse of this episode was a Sunday morning run in Yosemite Valley. I headed down the valley, enclosed by a high, lush, dark forest. A couple of hours into the run I turned a corner, and there before me, framed by the glorious forest, was the magnificence of El Capitan, illumined by brilliant sunlight. I felt that I had run directly into the pearly gates. The endorphins were bubbling over. Such an indelible experience recurs in all runners.

When to run can be important, but *where* is a trivial consideration. I recall an early-morning run around a lovely lake in Hanoi, where Senator John McCain's plane went down in 1967. I was obliviously taking in the site when I clumsily stumbled and fell comically face first into a puddle on the sidewalk. The crowd nearby doing their early-morning tai chi observed this crash bemusedly, what surely must have looked to them as an old guy running in his underpants, which interrupted their morning reverie as it did mine. But within an instant, we had all reclaimed our composure. It doesn't matter *how* you run, just as long as you do it.

Don't worry about your running style. I am a terrible runner, slow and awkward, and I feel as though I have army boots on. Style is not even a consideration. On my runs I am invariably passed by hordes of bikers coming and going. I occasionally hear their comments of derision. For a while I let these snide comments float by. "Why isn't that old buzzard at home in bed where he belongs?" For a while I was upset by such disdain for my effort, but now I have turned the argument around and reflect that their disapproval of my running is their problem, not mine. In adopting this perspective I rely on an unrecognized benefit of running: that it generates what the French call *sangfroid*, literally, cold blood, a supreme indifference to other callousness. So run for your *sangfroid*.

I run to finish. There is always a goal out there at the finish line of the marathon, 26 miles plus 385 yards from the starting line. I have started 40 marathons, the first in 1971, and finished 38 of them.

I dropped out in 1975 while running the Boston Marathon on a cold, miserable, wet day. When I reached the Newton hills just before Heartbreak Hill, I reasoned that our son Walter, age 16, had already finished in downtown Boston. And I could not rationalize keeping him chattering, waiting for his sluggard father for another two hours. So I bagged it.

The other non-finish happened in 2007 in Beijing. The run started at Mao's tomb in Tiananmen Square. First, past the Imperial Palace, and out into the boulevards of Beijing, past the governmental monoliths and future Olympic sites, initially cheered on by crowds, at least for a while. But one hour into the race the crowds had started to thin. By three hours I was alone. I approached the 13-mile halfway mark. The few officials confronted me to indicate that my run was over. The streets had been opened to traffic, and all the rest stations and directions had been removed. My run was only halfway through, I grumbled. What could I do about it? I'm an old white-haired anglo guy, running through the Chinese capital in his underpants. The only thing I recall of the taxi ride back to my hotel was the cabdriver's insistence on opening all the windows as my sneakers' aroma was disgusting.

One of the best parts of where we live is our close proximity to Stanford University. Nearby are patients, laureates, world experts in everything, noted authors, and cherished friends. Among these was Jack Barchas, in 1980 head of the Neurobiology Department at Stanford, now chief at Cornell. I mentioned to Jack that I was meeting a group of 100-mile trail runners in the Sierra Nevada mountains, doing what many regard as the toughest competitive run in the world. They may well be the fittest people in the world. Would it not be valuable to measure the endorphin levels in their blood? These magical molecules were held to be responsible for the runner's high, pain insensitivity, and other delights.

A few days later I found myself lugging a refrigerated centrifuge and blood-collecting gear up to the Sierras, where I collected blood samples from 51 of the runners before, during, and after their 100-mile runs. The "during" collection was the most fun, for I sat perched at the top of a 1,500-foot climb at mile 61 as the runners crested a ridge to provide me with a specimen.

After icing, spinning, and separating the samples, I sent them back to the Stanford lab. Jack measured the endorphin levels, which turned out to be the highest ever recorded. We reported these results in the *New England Journal of Medicine,* and ours was only the second publication on the effect of exercise on endorphins. The first was by fellow runner Leo Appenzeller in an obscure journal, lost now to the vagaries of history. I took these results and popularized them in a subsequent article I wrote for *Runner's World* magazine titled "The Runner's High."

Running is not only good for you, but it also makes you feel good, a positive addiction.

Stay high. I certainly plan to.

Even a "bad" run is better than no run at all. Running a little is better than not running at all. Every outing counts.

You never have a run that you regret. Don't feel like running? Do it anyway. You will always be glad you did.

There is no shame in walking occasionally.

Mix it up occasionally. Vary your routes. Vary your pace.

About breathing: Don't forget to exhale! Purge the CO_2 from your lungs consciously. Your body will reflexively make sure it's taking in enough oxygen, but you can help make the process efficient by consciously exhaling. Do abdominal breathing to get rid of side cramps or "stitches"—that is, consciously inhale from the lower part of your diaphragm.

There is no substitute for minutes, hours, days, and weeks on the trail or road. Running done right is joyous and addicting. You will never regret it.

A colleague sent me this ancient African proverb, which serves as a primal reminder:

Every morning in Africa.

A gazelle wakes up.

It knows it must outrun

the fastest lion,

or it will be killed.

Every morning in Africa

A lion wakes up,

It knows it must run faster

than the slowest gazelle

or it will starve

it doesn't matter whether

you're a lion or a gazelle.

When the sun comes up,

you'd better be running.

WALKING WORKS TOO

The directive to get out and walk seems to be a universal message, in the midst of an outright epidemic of obesity, indolence, and their cohorts, diabetes and all-around poor health. We can only reinforce the message. Walking is good; it's natural and should be encouraged at all times for all people.

Walking has demonstrable benefits, though it is not quite "running light." Running has a different energetic signature. In walking, one foot is always in contact with the ground. By definition, running requires both feet to be off the ground during each stride, which involves considerably more energy to push off one's entire weight. It is possible to run too much, thereby inviting injury and over-taxing one's resources. Walking, however, can occur in principle in an unlimited way, so long as one has the energy to continue putting one foot in front of the other. Most people don't walk nearly enough, but it's almost impossible to walk too much.

The admonition to walk has become almost a mantra for older people today. It should be equally (if not more so) promoted to children and young adults, for whom the risk of obesity and diabetes has longer and costlier consequences. Though the benefits of walking are widely taken for granted, there has been a scarcity of real data to support that theory in a quantifiable way.

Recently, however, 250,000 men and women in the 50 through 70 age range were subject to an intensive study exploring the relationship between a walking-based exercise program and life expectancy. All were put through exercise regimens designed by the American College of Sports Medicine in conjunction with the American Heart Association, titled *Exercise Guidelines for Healthy Adults and Exercise Guidelines for Adults Over 65.* The subjects represented a broad sample of body types and BMI ranges, and were put on a regimen of moderate exercise (brisk walking 30 minutes per day, five days per week) or intense exercise (20 minutes, three days per week). The results were clear and convincing. Those who engaged in the moderate walking program found their risk of death decreased by 27 percent. The vigorous exercise group saw in even larger benefit, 32 percent.

In an unexpected twist, overweight subjects got the same benefit from the same amount of exercise as the slimmer subjects, even if the person didn't lose weight during the study. In other words exercise trumps diet when it comes to health, a finding that runs counter to much of our accustomed thinking. This is an important insight, considering the emphasis on dietary factors in most public health discussions. As important as a healthy diet may be, a consistent exercise regimen will have a greater impact on our health.

Furthermore, the study found a significant reduction in deaths from heart disease among the exercisers, as well as a (somewhat lower) reduction in deaths from cancer.

Movement isn't always necessarily connected with formal or structured exercise, however. Unconscious activity can have a bearing as well, particularly those kinds of activities we usually associate with "fidgeting." The Mayo Clinic's Dr. James A. Levine has identified a category of activity called non-exercise activity thermogenesis (NEAT). We can think of this as spontaneous physical activity. In terms of physical energy expenditure, a very active person might account for up to 50 percent of his or her energy expenditure in NEAT calories. A very active person is someone who finds it hard to sit at a desk all day and is constantly finding reasons to get up and move around; the person who seems to be up and about most of the time and seems to have something in motion all the time. While this kind of movement is not as broadly effective a health strategy as formal exercise, it can have a positive bearing on metabolic maintenance. It all counts.

The movement imperative is the cornerstone of healthy aging. It means walking, running, exercising in any and all forms. It means doing. It means living!

INJURIES

Injuries can be the bane of exercise. Runners seem particularly susceptible, especially if one is running mostly on hard pavement. Toes, feet, ankles, knees, not to mention various muscles and tendons, all present opportunities for injury and pain. Weight training invites muscle tears and a host of tendon ailments. What to do?

In the first place, the obvious thing is to adopt conscious strategies designed to minimize opportunities for injury. For running these would include warming up before going full tilt. Warming up has several elements; it includes simply starting at a slower pace and slowly increasing your speed. Gentle stretching—not the full stretching that is best done *after* a workout—can help as well.

If something begins to hurt while you're running, pay attention. Misguided heroics have been the undoing of many a running program. Pain is your body's way of telling you that something is wrong. "Working through" the pain when it's associated with running is usually not a good idea. Working "around an injury," however, can be sound practice and a good way to avoid setbacks in your fitness.

Sometimes it may just be a matter of slowing down. Or walking. Or getting off your feet until the pain subsides.

Depending on the specifics of the injury, of course, the runner has a number of workout alternatives. Stationary bicycles have been a handy alternative to legions of hurt runners while they recuperate. In the 50-plus runner, plantar fasciitis, which causes excruciating heel pain, is becoming commonplace. The remedy involves daily stretching of the tendon and lots of time—and this is a great example of a time when a stationary bike can come in handy.

If you can walk, ramp up a walking regimen, keeping it under the pain threshold associated with running. Swimming is another worthy alternative.

Injuries are usually limited to a specific joint or limb. That means you don't necessarily have to stop exercising. Do other things. There are always optional exercises using ranges of motion that bypass an injury. Minor shoulder injuries, for instance, are common in the weight room. The shoulder is an amazingly complex joint, and a bit of tendinitis or a rotator cuff injury can threaten to throw you off entirely. But you will often find that the injury is a problem only in a very specific range of motion, and the shoulder may still be perfectly capable of a number of exercises that don't bother it at all. The guiding principle of "know thyself" is enormously useful in dealing with injuries. It will help you develop an accurate sense of what requires medical attention, what requires simple rest, and what can be "worked around."

Every active person sustains occasional minor injuries along the way. But if we pay attention, we don't necessarily have to stop because of our injuries; we can merely slow down or shift routines. Best of all, our bodies are amazing healing machines, and the more fit we are, the faster and better we recuperate from injury.

THE COMPONENTS OF SUCCESSFUL AGING

We can now propose the essential components of a life program that maximizes our potential not only to live to 100 (or beyond) but also to enjoy the full measure of living—in a healthy, functional, capable way—that our evolutionary heritage has equipped us for. Here are the essential components of a healthy, long life:

- *Lean muscle mass.* Our skeletal muscles are the principal drivers of our metabolic engine. The ratio of lean muscle mass to total body weight is a key health metric.

- *VO$_2$max.* This is a measure of the body's ability to transport and utilize oxygen during exercise. It is considered the best indicator of cardiorespiratory endurance, and is widely accepted as the single best measure of cardiovascular fitness and aerobic power.

- *Nutrition.* It has been said that "You are what you eat." While that's not quite as true as many would like, what we consume (and how much of it) is perhaps the most controversial topic in health and longevity today. And that includes the multibillion dollar industries of vitamins and nutritional supplements, which is justifiably controversial as a factor in personal health strategies.

- *Sex.* It is remarkable that the subject of sex is so infrequently encountered in the larger discussion of longevity and aging-related health matters. We are accustomed to regular advisories to the effect that age should be no deterrent to an active sex life; what we rarely see is a deep and analytical reflection on the elemental relationship between sex and life. Sex and sexuality are—or should be—directly linked to the forces and phenomena that define youth, vitality, and life itself.

- *A healthy brain.* There are two dimensions to this factor. One is the physical health of our central processor, its cellular vitality and function. The other is our psychic state, that complex array of attitude, desire, will, and adaptability that we sometimes label "the intangibles," and that can enhance or subvert the other factors. Stress, for example, can literally kill.

- *Engagement*—being necessary. Perhaps the most common factor among known centenarians is the presence of strong social bonds, deeply rooted relationships, and/or some form of active engagement that provides a passion for facing each day anew. This cannot be overstated.

- *Movement* is the crux, the essence of expressing life as purposeful beings. It is both cause and effect, an enabler of health and the result of health. Muscle gives us the strength to move and the capability to perform the functions that express our aliveness; oxygen provides the fuel for movement and the combustive force that drives our cells; nutrition provides continuity as well as energy; the healthy brain gives us the internal milieu that invests our lives with value, our sense of self; sex and engagement ensure that our circle of health encompasses not just our bodies but our interconnectedness with others of our species. It is a remarkable constellation of tools from which we can build our path to 100 healthy years.

CHAPTER 4

AEROBIC FITNESS:
THE CRITICAL PATH

OXYGEN—THE FUEL OF LIFE

The human body is nearly two-thirds oxygen. The fact that oxygen is also the most abundant element in the earth's crust, making up nearly 50 percent of it, is an almost poetic reminder that we are literally "of the earth." Historically, oxygen, or its absence, has been the key determinant for life on the planet. Earth's early atmosphere contained negligible oxygen, and for good reason; it is one of the most reactive of all elements. Free oxygen atoms will seek other elements to combine with, such as hydrogen, to form water, or iron to form rust, or carbon to make carbon dioxide. Two billion years ago, the first photosynthetic organisms began using sunlight to convert water and carbon dioxide into molecular oxygen, gifting the planet with atmospheric oxygen in relative abundance, igniting the evolutionary firestorm that led to the proliferation of life forms we know today.

The generation and maintenance of all our life processes are driven by four basic factors: carbohydrates, water, proteins, and energy. Oxygen can be thought of as the overriding key ingredient in all four of these life-enabling components. Every day we breathe, on average, 20,000 times. Oxygen enters our body as molecules of two coupled oxygen atoms. It leaves the body in one of two ways: as two oxygen atoms attached to a carbon atom (carbon dioxide), or as one oxygen atom bonded to two hydrogen atoms as water. In between, oxygen is the essential component enabling the metabolic functions of the body. The oxygen concentration in a healthy human body is approximately three times that of air, our fundamental fuel source.

All metabolic processes in the body are regulated by oxygen. Even our abilities to think, feel, and act require oxygen-related energy production. Oxygen plays a vital role in proper metabolic functions, blood circulation, digestion, the assimilation of nutrients, and the elimination of cellular and metabolic wastes. Sufficient oxygen helps the body in its ability to rebuild itself and maintain a sound immune system. In what we can think of as an inverse priority rule, it has been suggested that the most important health factors are those we can least live without. For instance, one can actually exist without food for about 40 days. Without water, we are good for about seven days at most. Without oxygen, however, life ceases to exist in a matter of minutes.

All of this underscores the critical role that aerobic fitness plays in our health, wellness, and life span. By definition, aerobic exercise is brisk physical activity that requires the heart and lungs to work harder to meet the body's increased oxygen demand. Aerobic exercise increases the amount of oxygen available to the blood, as well as increases the circulation of blood throughout our body, delivering more oxygen to all our vital organs. In addition, consistent aerobic exercise will cause our blood vessels, particularly our coronary artery, to increase in size and efficiency, phenotypic plasticity at work! Duration of exercise is important. To gain full aerobic benefit, the activity should be sustained for 20 to 60 minutes each session.

Some examples of widely accessible aerobic exercises include cycling/biking, running, swimming, cross-country skiing, playing basketball, jumping rope, skating, walking briskly, and many forms of dancing. In addition to these activities, you can get an aerobic workout through stationary exercise machines such as cycles, treadmills, stair-climbers, and rowing machines.

THE RESPIRATORY PROCESS

As air moves into the lungs, small sacs called alveoli are inflated. Capillaries surround each sac and force the red blood cells to flow nearly single file while each blood cell exchanges its load of carbon dioxide for a fresh charge of oxygen. From the lungs, the oxygen is transported by arterial blood to every cell in the body. In the tissues of the body, the blood cells again pass through another series of capillaries where they drop off oxygen and pick up carbon dioxide for their return trip to the lungs.

The general process that cells use to turn food into energy is called respiration. Respiration is the opposite of photosynthesis. What plants do in photosynthesis to convert energy into sugar, respiration does in reverse to change sugar into energy. Within the cell, this operation is driven by a circular sequence called the Krebs cycle. This process stores energy in a molecule called adenosine triphosphate (ATP). The operation ultimately uses oxygen to combust glucose, and creates carbon dioxide and water by-products according to this classic chemical formula:

$$C_6H_{12}O_6 + 6O_2 \rightarrow 6CO_2 + 6H_2O + ATP$$

This formula is to cellular biology what Einstein's famous $E = mc^2$ is to nuclear energy, a fundamental description of the conversion of matter to energy.

It is the presence of oxygen that allows the body to convert food to energy. This happens essentially the same way in nerves, muscles, the heart, and all body tissues. When deprived of oxygen, cellular respiration eventually comes to a halt, and the cells will die.

A liter of blood can dissolve 200 cc of oxygen gas, which is much more than water can dissolve. If blood is, indeed, thicker than water, it's due to the dense concentration of oxygen. After being carried in blood to a body tissue in need of oxygen, O_2 is handed off to an enzyme that uses this oxygen to combust the fuel that drives our metabolism. Carbon dioxide, a waste product, is released from the cell and into the blood, where it combines with bicarbonate and hemoglobin for transport to the lungs. Blood circulates back to the lungs, and the process repeats.

The critical role of oxygen can be dramatically seen in the operation of the brain. The brain is an especially demanding organ, processing billions of bits of information each second. Though it represents only 2 percent of the human body weight, it receives 20 percent of total body oxygen consumption (as well as 15 percent of the cardiac output and 25 percent of total body glucose utilization).

The energy consumption for the brain to simply survive is 0.1 calories per minute, while this value can be as high as 1.5 calories per minute during concentrated problem solving. When neurons in a particular region of the brain are highly active, they accelerate the consumption of oxygen, which results in the demand for extra blood flow to that region. Degenerative diseases, such as Alzheimer's disease, Parkinson's disease, motor neuron disease, and Huntington's disease, are associated with the gradual death of individual neurons, in which oxygen deprivation plays a central role, leading to compromised movement control, memory, and cognition.

Mental performance in the human body can be improved by "feeding" the brain extra oxygen or glucose, according to research published recently that could have implications for the treatment of dementia. A decrease in the oxygen supply to the brain creates conditions like tiredness, depression, irritability, poor judgment, and a variety of health problems. Increasing the oxygen supply to the brain and nervous system can remedy these conditions.

The amount of oxygen used up at the cellular level during exercise is referred to as oxygen uptake. In other words, it's the central measure of how we use oxygen effectively to support, sustain, and extend our life processes. It is well established now that both moderate and vigorous body movement along with the associated muscle work increase oxygen demand in the cells. Muscular activity accelerates the rate of oxygen uptake from the blood. Regular body movement, and the increased rate of breathing that goes with it, cause increased functional efficiency in the uptake and utilization of oxygen from the blood.

The Framingham Heart Study, a landmark investigation begun in 1948, tracked a group of adults for decades to identify the common factors associated with cardiovascular disease. Among the findings was a distinct correlation between decreased respiratory capacity and increased mortality. Other studies seeking similar data followed. In Australia, an extensive 13-year study concluded that respiratory capacity was a powerful determining variable of longevity. In fact, the study demonstrated a higher correlation of respiratory capacity to life span than any other variable, including tobacco use, insulin metabolism, and cholesterol levels.

Aerobic capacity is the term commonly used when discussing oxygen usage associated with exercise. VO_2max is a measure of oxygen consumption at the point of maximum exertion and is an important metric for competitive athletes. Not surprisingly, athletic pursuits with the highest cardiovascular demands produce the highest VO_2max scores. For instance, the highest known scores were taken from competitive Nordic skiers.

Although VO_2max is not typically a concern for the average citizen, the concept is important to understand. We have a specific capacity to provide oxygen to our tissues through our cardiorespiratory system. Increasing our VO_2max is a direct means of ensuring that our bodily tissues that are required to do work, to support us, to keep all of our components active and functioning optimally, are getting all the fuel they require. Maximizing our ability to supply oxygen to keep our tissues nourished is essential to achieving peak health..

Our VO_2max normally decreases with age. Typically, the decline is around 1 percent per year or 10 percent per decade after the age of 25. However, this deterioration does not have to be a *fait accompli*. A number of studies have shown that previously sedentary people, put on a program of training at 75 percent of aerobic capacity for 30 minutes, three times a week for just six months, have registered on average a 15 percent to 20 percent increase in their VO_2max. Once again, the message is clear and compelling: It is never too late to start exercising, and always too soon to stop!

Athletes who have very high scores in their prime, and then become sedentary, find that their VO_2max will revert to that of a sedentary person. But "master" athletes who maintain a consistent level of activity throughout their adult life are able to maintain much of their youthful capacity, losing VO_2max at a rate of less than half a percent per year. It's hard to imagine a more convincing demonstration of the "use it or lose it" rule.

The perceptive reader may note that oxygen is also the source of free radicals, those ionized molecules that occur as a by-product of normal cell metabolism. If we introduce more oxygen into our system through exercise, shouldn't that exacerbate the production of even more free radicals? No. Any increase in free radicals is more than compensated for by the additional production of enzymes and other molecular compounds (like hydrogen peroxide, H_2O_2) that scavenge those harmful age-accelerating molecules.

Free radicals occupy much of the attention of researchers who study aging, and have spawned an enormous industry in antioxidant remedies. We will look at these in depth in subsequent chapters.

We all breathe, whether we want to or not. Ability to hold one's breath, a skill with only a handful of uses, is measured in mere minutes at best. But thinking about how we breathe can be useful in several ways. Competitive athletes are very aware of their breathing, and the need to optimize the volume of oxygen they can deliver through the lungs, as well as how to most efficiently get rid of the CO_2 by-product. One doesn't have to be an athlete, however, to benefit from thinking about the connection between conscious breathing and physical exertion.

Though not everyone agrees on the same principle of breathing, most concur that it is generally considered good practice to breathe through both the mouth and the nose. The act of methodically breathing through both the nostrils and the mouth can result in more oxygen passing through the airways. Oxygen should come from the diaphragm and not the chest. If the breathing is done correctly, you should feel your stomach contract in and out. If it is done incorrectly, you may add extra strain to your shoulders, resulting in a tighter feel in the upper body. This can of course have adverse effects, forcing you to make your run a shorter one.

Another widely accepted practice of breathing techniques while running is maintaining what is known as a breathing ratio. A breathing ratio of 3:2 can help keep a healthy supply of oxygen circulating in the body. Keeping the 3:2 ratio means that for the first three steps you're inhaling, then exhaling for the next two, alternating between steps, as shown in Table 4.1.

A 3:2 ratio is most commonly used for a light jog. If you are running exceptionally fast, your body may instinctively switch to a 2:1 ratio. That means for every two steps of inhaling, you only exhale for one step.

Table 4.1

Footstrike	Breathing Pattern
Left	Inhale
Right	Inhale
Left	Inhale
Right	Exhale
Left	Exhale
Right	Inhale
Left	Inhale
Right	Inhale
Left	Exhale
Right	Exhale

EFFECTS OF AEROBIC FITNESS

There is simply no one therapeutic remedy better for enforcing optimum health and improving your longevity prospects than consistent aerobic fitness. The list of benefits associated with increasing one's aerobic fitness is long and compelling. They include:

- Improving the function of the heart. Enlarging the arteries through aerobic conditioning is one of our best examples of phenotypic plasticity.
- Strengthening muscles, ligaments, tendons, and joints.
- Improving blood pressure control. In particular, it lowers high blood pressure.
- Increasing the high-density lipoprotein (HDL), that is, the "good" cholesterol, in the blood.
- Lowering the triglyceride levels (fatty substances) in the blood.
- Assisting in weight control, by reducing body fat.
- Alleviating muscle pain and improving walking capability in people who suffer from peripheral arterial disease.
- Reducing the rate of occurrence of various types of cancer, particularly of the colon, breast, prostate, and lungs.
- Preventing osteoporosis.
- Preventing lower back pain in many cases.

- Reducing the incidence of stroke.

- Improving the functioning of the immune system.

- Decreasing the insulin requirement and improving glucose control in type 1 (insulin-dependent) diabetes; preventing the development of type 2 (non-insulin-dependent) diabetes, and improving glucose tolerance if this condition exists.

- Assisting in the control of joint pain and swelling in people who suffer from arthritis.

- Improving temperature regulation at rest and during exercise in different environments.

Aerobic fitness is a very important factor in growth and development during childhood and adolescence as well as a critical factor in the aging process. A high level of aerobic conditioning during the growing years is the best way to ensure full development of the muscles, bones, and cardiorespiratory system. Aerobic exercise is more important in this respect than body weight. Since aerobic fitness is a measure of the ability to sustain prolonged efforts, it determines the degree of fatigue that almost everybody experiences in daily life. The higher your aerobic fitness, the less fatigue you experience, and the more quickly you will be able to recover from it.

In advancing age, aerobic fitness provides a particularly critical metric of one's "molecular age" as opposed to chronological age. As we have seen earlier, a 70-year-old individual who exhibits good aerobic fitness may actually have the equivalent of 40-year-old cardiorespiratory, muscular, and other bodily systems. This "effective age" offset towers over every other remedial claim by anti-aging products, which, at best, suggest three to seven years of extended life—and invariably without consideration of the quality of those additional years. Aerobic fitness is unquestionably the best and most definitive marker of overall health and potential life span.

As a shield against the major disease threats of aging, aerobic fitness is unparalleled. We can examine how it works to prevent heart disease, stroke, and cancer.

Heart Disease.

A Japanese study performed at the University of Tsukuba Institute of Clinical Medicine surveyed 33 different fitness studies, covering nearly 190,000 people, to determine the effect of aerobic fitness on mortality, and determined that those with a low fitness level had a 70 percent higher risk of death from any cause compared with those with a high fitness level. The correlation was so convincing that researchers concluded that aerobic fitness levels could be used as a reliable predictor of heart disease.

Cardiorespiratory fitness is measured through exercise stress testing, in which participants typically exercise by walking on a treadmill until they become fatigued or exhausted. Fitness level is then estimated as maximal aerobic capacity expressed in metabolic equivalents (METs).

METs indicate the amount of oxygen the body consumes during activity and represents a standard scale on which to measure exercise workload. One MET is equivalent to the oxygen the body uses at rest. Being able to attain a high degree of oxygen use during exercise, and therefore have a high MET level, is an indicator of physical fitness.

The researchers found that, compared to those at the higher-level scores, those with low cardiorespiratory fitness had a 70 percent higher risk of death from any cause and a 56 percent higher risk of fatal heart disease. Compared to those with an intermediate level of physical fitness, those with relatively low scores had a 40 percent higher risk of death from any cause and a 47 percent higher risk of death from heart disease. Some fitness is unequivocally better than none!

The researchers concluded that a minimal level of cardiorespiratory fitness of 7.9 METs may be important for overall health. Expressed in terms of walking speed, men around 50 years of age should be able to walk at a continuous speed of four miles per hour and women should be able to walk three miles per hour, on level ground, or be able to complete at least six minutes of a standard treadmill stress test (which involves walking up an incline, but at a slower pace).

They found even a one-MET increase in aerobic fitness was associated with a 13 percent lower risk of death from any cause and a 15 percent lower risk of heart disease. To put that in perspective, the difference between riding a golf cart and walking while playing golf is one MET level.

Another study by the Preventive Medicine Research Lab at the Pennington Biomedical Research Center at Louisiana State University in Baton Rouge, Louisiana, sought to find how to get people exercising who had aversions to it. They enlisted 500 women ages 45 to 75, many of them retired teachers. All of them had become overweight and were living sedentary lives. Most of them were also unaware that the leading cause of death in women is cardiovascular disease, and that postmenopausal women were at much higher risk.

Researchers wanted to determine exactly *how much* exercise is sufficient to protect older women who have not made physical activity a priority. To answer this question, volunteers were divided into two groups. One group of women was instructed to walk on a treadmill three times a week for about 25 minutes at a time. Others were instructed to ride a stationary bike or walk on a treadmill for three hours per week. All of the subjects had their heart rate monitored and were instructed to keep their workouts to a modest intensity. The target training intensity was 50 percent of each woman's peak aerobic capacity.

To their surprise, the investigators found a sharp rise in fitness of the first group that exercised only 75 minutes per week, and moderately at that. At the end of the six-month study, though none of the women lost significant weight or saw a drop in blood pressure, all of the women had noticeably improved their aerobic fitness. They were able to move longer and faster without becoming winded.

Studies like these have led to the broad conclusion that aerobic fitness alone is a key predictor of longevity. It doesn't matter whether the individual loses weight or has other risk factors associated with disease. Increasing fitness, even a little bit, clearly reduces the chances of heart attack and other major causes of mortality.

The Louisiana study also found that the more exercise women did, the better off they were in terms of fitness. Women who biked or walked on treadmills for three hours per week ended up about twice as fit as those who exercised for just 71 minutes a week. It is easy to conclude that one does not have to exercise a lot in order to begin seeing results. And that increasing the amount of exercise increases the degree of fitness in proportion.

Stroke

Another large, long-running study supported by the American Heart Association has suggested that a moderate level of aerobic fitness can result in a significant reduction of stroke risk in both men and women. This study, conducted by the Prevention Research Center at the University of South Carolina, tracked a group of more than 60,000 people for 30 years, between 1970 and 2001.

Fitness has a protective effect regardless of the presence or absence of other stroke risk factors, including family history of cardiovascular disease, diabetes, high blood pressure, elevated cholesterol levels, and obesity. This study is the first to suggest that there may be a significant independent association between cardiorespiratory fitness and fatal and nonfatal stroke in men and nonfatal stroke in women.

Stroke is often fatal, and claims about 150,000 lives each year; it's the number three cause of death in the United States. Data was analyzed from more than 60,000 who participated in the Aerobics Center Longitudinal Study between 1970 and 2001 at the Cooper Aerobics Center in Dallas. The participants ranged from 18 to 100 years old, and all were free of known cardiovascular diseases when they began the study. They were followed for an average of 18 years, and in this time, 863 people, 692 men and 171 women, had strokes.

When they began the study, each participant underwent a test to measure cardiorespiratory fitness: They walked on a treadmill at increasing grade and/or speed until they reached the limits of their aerobic capacity.

Men in the top quartile (25th percentile) of fitness had a 40 percent lower relative risk of stroke compared to men in the lowest quartile. This inverse relationship remained after adjusting for other factors such as smoking, alcohol intake, family history of cardiovascular disease, body mass index, high blood pressure, diabetes, and high cholesterol levels.

In the case of women, those in the higher fitness percentiles had a 43 percent lower relative risk than those in the lowest fitness level.

It was observed that the overall stroke risk dropped substantially at the moderate fitness level, with the protective effect continuing almost unchanged through higher fitness levels. That is equivalent to 30 minutes or more of brisk walking, or an equal aerobic activity, five days a week.

It was concluded that a low-to-moderate amount of aerobic fitness for men and women across the whole adult age spectrum would be enough to substantially reduce stroke risk. Although stroke death rates have declined over the past few decades, the public health burden of stroke-related disabilities continues to be large and may even increase in coming years, as the population ages.

Cancer

Rigorous research into the relationship between aerobic fitness and cancer has only appeared in recent years. Nonetheless, the results so far have ranged from encouraging to impressive. The molecular biochemistry of cancer puts it in quite a different category from heart disease and stroke, but it is possible nonetheless to connect the dots in many cases and see how aerobic factors, whether a sufficiency or deficiency of aerobic fitness, are linked to carcinogenesis.

Breast, colon, and prostate cancers, three of the most common cancers, have been studied in the context of aerobic fitness and found to have specific correlations. For example, men who engage in at least four hours of moderate to vigorous aerobic exercise a week can significantly reduce their risk of colon cancer, according to a report from the first randomized clinical trial to test the effect of exercise on colon-cancer biomarkers in colon tissue. Colon cancer is particularly of concern in the context of aging—around 90 percent of all cases occur in people 50 and older. Aerobic exercise at this level reduces a specific risk factor—rapid cellular proliferation associated with the formation of colon polyps and colon cancer in men. Men who met the study's exercise prescription of an hour of aerobic activity per day, six days a week, for a year saw a substantial decrease in the amount of cellular proliferation in the areas of the colon that are most vulnerable to colon cancer.

It was also found that even four hours of exercise weekly was enough to produce a significant benefit. Specifically, at that rate, the researchers saw a decrease in the number of actively dividing cells, or cellular proliferation, in the lining of the colon, or epithelium, which helps regulate the absorption of water and nutrients.

Body weight did not appear to have an impact on the effect of exercise on cellular proliferation. The study showed that the effects were independent of the weight of the subject. Vigorous exercise yielded measurable benefits for men of any size, so long as they worked out nearly every day.

Breast cancer has seen a number of encouraging studies as well. In one, researchers tracked 65,000 nurses aged 24 to 42 and found that women who started exercising as young as 12 years old received protective benefits from breast cancer when older, and that both young girls and middle-aged women can reduce cancer risk by exercising. Women who were physically active as teens and young adults were 23 percent less likely to develop post-menopausal breast cancer than sedentary women.

More recently, a landmark study at the Cooper Institute, under Dr. Steven Blair, analyzed more than 14,000 women in what was claimed to be the first study to evaluate the association of objectively measured fitness and risk of death from breast cancer. The results were unambiguous: Women with moderate or high aerobic fitness levels were much less likely to die from breast cancer. On the other hand, women in the study's lowest fitness category were nearly *three times more likely* to die from breast cancer than women in the most fit group.

This was the first study to examine the relationship between objectively measured fitness (where subjects' fitness routines are monitored rather than self-reported) and risk of succumbing to breast cancer. The results revealed a stronger protective effect from exercise than could have been inferred from previous studies that relied on data reported by the subjects, leading researchers to believe that their conclusions were particularly validated.

The researchers studied women from 20 to 83 years of age who had no previous history of breast cancer. The study participants submitted to maximal exercise tests on a treadmill, between 1973 and 2001, and were monitored for breast cancer mortality through 2003. Women who did a minimum of 150 minutes of moderate-intensity activity per week, including walking, escaped the low fitness category. Further, it was found that this moderate-intensity activity can be accumulated in ten-minute bouts. This level of exercise meets the U.S. Department of Health & Human Services' *Physical Activity Guidelines for Americans* recommendations, and can be easily achieved in 30 minutes of exercise five days a week.

To develop the highest fitness category in this study, Blair said, women should aim for the "high activity" level recommended by federal guidelines, which includes 300 minutes of moderate-intensity activity, such as walking, over the course of the week. This can be achieved through 150 minutes/week of more vigorous activity, such as jogging or aerobics classes.

More than 40,000 women die each year from breast cancer. Finding a strong association between cancer avoidance and fitness, which can be improved by the relatively inexpensive lifestyle commitment of regular physical activity, suggests a powerful mandate, the absolute necessity of aerobic conditioning. In addition, not surprisingly, the study found that women with high aerobic fitness had lower body mass index, better cholesterol levels, lower blood pressure, and fewer chronic conditions such as diabetes and cardiovascular disease.

Prostate cancer will strike around 200,000 men in the United States this year. Although mortality rates are relatively low compared to other forms of cancer, the lifestyle consequences of prostate cancer can be profound. Yet, it too appears amenable to an exercise regimen as a prevention strategy. The Cooper Clinic study cited earlier analyzed 13,000 men over an 18-year period. The conclusion: Moderate to high levels of aerobic fitness yield statistically significant results against the incidence of prostate cancer. As little as 1,000 calories per week of exercise (equivalent to walking 30 minutes a day, five days per week) reduced the risk in the study group. At least part of the beneficial effect can likely be attributed to the fact that exercise lowers testosterone levels during the periods of exertion, and that periodic suppression can make a difference. Those who exercised at high levels, around 4,000 calories per week, showed a marked improvement. A subsequent Harvard study showed men who exercised "very frequently" had only half the incidence of prostate cancer as those with little or no exercise.

In a study at Duke University reported in the *Journal of Urology* researchers found that among 190 men who underwent biopsies to detect possible prostate cancer, those who regularly exercised were less likely to be diagnosed with the disease. Men who exercised moderately—the equivalent of three or more hours of brisk walking per week—were two-thirds less likely than their sedentary counterparts to have prostate cancer. Among those who did have cancer, men who reported as little as one hour of walking per week were less likely to have aggressive, faster-growing cancer. Regular exercise remained linked to a lower risk of prostate cancer even after the researchers factored in a number of other variables—including age, weight, race, and the presence of any other medical conditions.

To be clear, there are no guarantees that exercise will prevent cancer, heart disease, or stroke. Life holds few such guarantees under any circumstance. What does matter is that we can substantially influence the probability that we will be afflicted. We are all unconscious statisticians, intuitively computing, in the back of our mind, the odds of outcomes that concern us as we go through our daily routines. Unless we have some pathological deficiency, we know that when we choose to pull out of the flow of traffic to pass another car, our odds of remaining safe are taking a momentary dip. By the same token, we usually know when we are increasing the risk on our well-being, and have some form of mental activity that tries to steer us onto a safer course. The more knowledge we have of unfavorable consequences, the better we become at those intuitive calculations, and the better equipped we are to make good decisions about our health. And we will live longer.

Fitness is not a guarantee, but it is overwhelmingly favored by the oddsmakers. It is the classic fate vs. choice dilemma. We can rest assured in the knowledge that if we pursue a sound life program of ongoing fitness, the odds of avoiding life-threatening illnesses are on our side. And if we don't, we are simply defaulting, throwing ourselves at the mercy of chance.

CHAPTER 5

FIT AND FUNCTIONAL:
MUSCLE AND MOVEMENT

As a culture, we have a long history of uncomfortable associations with muscle. For a long time, muscles were associated with people who did hard labor, the working class. It was considered a mark of success or class distinction when one didn't have to be physically strong. In recent times, building of muscle was looked down upon as a kind of unsavory vanity. There were the bodybuilders, a fringe culture who were regarded as oddities and who were suspect in other ways as a result of their fitness fetish. It simply wasn't "normal" to be muscular. In today's world, we seem to have gone overboard in another direction. Our popular culture icons often come with ridiculously showy musculature, trying to match comic book characters with impossible physiques bordering on the grotesque.

We are just now beginning to fully appreciate the relationship of our muscle structure to the full spectrum of our health and our potential for longevity. There are three basic considerations here. The first is strength, because physical strength is the antidote to frailty. The second is the relationship of muscle to metabolic function, our "youth engine." And the third is the role of lean muscle mass as a safeguard against injury and disease.

STRENGTH—THE IMPORTANCE OF MUSCLE

Are you strong enough to live to 100? Frailty, the great bane of aging, is, more than anything, a loss of physical strength generally associated with the wasting away of muscle tissue. Maintaining sufficient muscle strength to conduct the routines of daily life comfortably and safely should be a minimum requirement for everyone. To be able to move, to lift, to push, to carry things, to maintain one's balance and avoid accidents.

Sarcopenia, a term derived from the Greek words for "vanishing flesh," is the gradual loss of lean muscle tissue associated with aging. A few decades ago this condition did not even have a name, but with an increasingly aging population, it is now well on the way to becoming as familiar a word as osteoporosis. Responsible for robbing both women and men of their strength, health, mobility, and independence in their senior years, sarcopenia is a significant global health problem and is one of the most serious long-term threats to independent living as adults age. Seen most prominently in physically inactive people, sarcopenia exerts its debilitating effects in a slow, barely perceptible fashion over a period of decades.

The loss of muscle begins at around the age of 30 at the rate of 10 percent per decade, increasing to 15 percent per decade as people reach their sixties and seventies, and then about 30 percent per decade thereafter. This insidious process, left to its own devices, robs people of their functional health and mobility and further pushes them into unhealthy and inactive lifestyles. The vicious cycle continues with increasing risk of other diseases associated with inactivity.

Again, we refer back to the Disuse Syndrome and discover that all is not what it seems to be.

Several studies have shown that muscle wasting is attributable to the fact that older people seem to be less able to convert food into muscle tissue. This has mostly to do with the release of insulin that slows the breakdown of muscle tissue after eating. Testing on subjects at the University of Nottingham showed that younger subjects responded to direct injection of insulin into leg muscles, but older subjects didn't. Further examination found a direct correspondence with blood flow to the muscles. That is, the older group had a much smaller rate of blood flow to the affected areas. Following up this initial study, the older group began an exercise regimen with weights, three times per week for a period of 20 weeks. At the end of that period, they had completely reversed the wasting effects, and had restored blood flow to the legs to the same level as the younger group!

A similar investigation was undertaken by researchers from the University of Texas Medical Branch at Galveston. They injected two groups of men, one with an average age of 28 and the other with an average age of 70, with amino acids (insulin normally drives amino acids into muscles to help them recover from exercise and maintain their size), and then tracked the rate of muscle breakdown. They found that muscle breakdown followed the same pattern in both groups, or that the capability of the muscle tissue itself was no different. The conclusion: The altered exercise and diet patterns of the older subjects was to blame for muscle breakdown, not the age of their muscle tissue.

This is a profoundly significant finding, that muscle tissue has the ability to continue to respond and regenerate more or less indefinitely as we grow older. At Tufts University, a group of frail, elderly people were put through a weight training regimen where, with each exercise, they performed eight repetitions of each routine with a weight at 80 percent of the amount they could lift one time. These sessions were repeated three times per week. On average, the subjects gained strength at the rate of 5 percent per training day, a remarkable performance and a testament to our inherent elasticity. A number of other research studies have shown that untrained elderly people can experience substantial strength gains after as little as two weeks of moderate weight training.

All of this is good news, of course, to those who are well into middle age and beyond, and have not been systematically active to this point. But it should be an admonition to those in the first half of their years. The lesson is simple: Create a healthy, strong body early and then simply maintain it. It is much easier to maintain than to build when you are in your later years. It is never too soon to start. In fact, a study conducted by South Dakota State University determined that children with higher proportions of lean muscle mass also had the strongest bones and better overall growth performance.

HOW TO

Today, there are gyms and health clubs galore. Gyms are convenient to be sure, but if you can't find one, that's no excuse for avoiding a healthy regimen of training. To train at a level that will keep a person strong, active, and energized indefinitely requires no heroics. Let's proceed by simply answering the most obvious questions.

How much time should I devote to resistance training?

Thirty to 40 minutes, three times a week, would be ample time to do everything one could hope to achieve, short of Olympic ambitions.

What should I be doing?

Think of your major muscle groups. In each of them there is a principle of opposition: For every push muscle there is a pull muscle, and a
training routine should address each one. Think arms, shoulders, chest,
back, abdominals, legs. If you have a cardio routine with running, hiking, or biking, it can be argued that you don't even need to do leg workouts with weights. But it's good to do something with your legs if for no
other reason than to affirm your leg strength objectively by knowing
that you can handle specific amounts of resistance. Here's an example of
a complete workout that you can do in 30 minutes:

Two sets of chest presses

One set of bicep curls

One set of lateral raises

Two sets of seated rows

Two sets of pull-downs

Two sets of abdominal crunches

One set of back extensions

One set of leg presses

That's 12 separate exercise routines. If one worked in two-and-a-
half-minute intervals, you could do it all in 30 minutes and have plenty
of time to catch your breath, get a drink of water, and even socialize a bit
in between.

Only two sets? I thought it was supposed to be three.

Recent studies have shown that a person can get full benefit from two sets rather than three, so long as a sufficient amount of weight is used.

How do I know how much weight I should use?

We are all stronger than we give ourselves credit for. We should strive to avoid injury, of course, but we should also use sufficient resistance to maximize our muscles' response to stimuli. If you have little or no prior experience, you should start out with light weights. But it's easy to find out what an optimum weight should be. Can you do 15 repetitions (reps, in gym parlance) with the weight you have selected for a specific exercise? Then it's too light. Ideally, you should use a weight that you can do 8 to 10 reps with, and the last rep should take some effort and concentration. If it's too easy, it's your body's way of telling you to add more weight, that it can't "hear" you yet.

When you can do more than ten easily, it's time to add weight incrementally. If you are consistent, over time you will find your ability to add weight to your routines beginning to taper off. We all have a natural limit unique to our body type, size, and DNA. Once we've approached those limits, it's a simple matter to maintain. And as we've shown, the evidence is mounting that one can maintain near-peak strength indefinitely.

What if I have no reasonable access to a gym and can't have weights at home?

Be inventive. Be resourceful. Every routine listed above can be done with a six-foot length of surgical tubing tied off on a doorknob or other secure points around the house.

Aren't there significant differences between men and women when it comes to strength training and weight lifting? Shouldn't there be separate guidelines for women?

Yes, there are gender differences, but they are not particularly important. Testosterone is a factor in muscle development and power. On average, women have about 10 percent the testosterone level of men. What that means is that most women will never gain the massive amounts of muscle that male bodybuilders do, no matter how much weight training they might do. Otherwise, it's a non-issue. Generally, women are reported to have 40 percent to 60 percent of the upper body strength of men and 70 percent to 75 percent of the lower body strength, largely because men are, on average, simply bigger than women and have broader frames to accommodate greater muscle mass. What is really important from a health and longevity standpoint is the proportion of lean muscle mass to overall body weight. And in those terms, on the basis of strength to lean muscle-mass ratios, women are equal to men. All the advisories about workout techniques apply equally to both sexes.

What of the danger of losing my flexibility when I gain muscle?

Actually, you are more likely to gain flexibility when you work out with weights than to lose it, especially if you follow a routine that involves all the major muscle groups as outlined earlier. The real danger is that, as we age, we tend to limit ourselves to efficient patterns of movement and fall into limited and restrictive types. This leads to chronic, self-imposed limitations on our range of motion. As a result, small supporting muscles atrophy, forcing other systems to take over their normal functions. The results can include chronic pain, joint problems, and a broad range of symptoms of aging.

TUNING THE METABOLIC ENGINE WITH LEAN MUSCLE MASS

Metabolism is measured in calories, a basic unit of heat. It's a measure of how much energy is actually being expended in maintaining our bodily functions. Every body contains both muscle tissue and fat tissue, both of which are part of our metabolic cycle. While we are at rest, all of our internal functions operate at a basal rate, or what is called resting metabolism. While it is sometimes claimed that fat is simply "dead weight" with no metabolic value, that's not quite true. Fat does generate metabolic activity, though at a much lower level than muscle. It is estimated that the basal rate of fat metabolism is about two calories per pound. Muscle tissue, on the other hand, consumes six to ten calories at rest and a great deal more when active.

The logic is simple and straightforward. Even if we haven't an inkling of the biochemistry involved, we are all basically aware of our metabolism because we experience it in our sense of daily energy and we refer to it casually as something we tend to associate in a positive way with our youth. What too many people have not understood or intuited is that metabolism is not hard-wired; it is driven in large measure by the energetic signals we induce by our behavior patterns.

Obesity is a metabolism killer. The intricate linkage between metabolism and the broad network of bodily functions yields a clue to why obesity is associated with so many other contemporary health issues. And it further underscores the importance of sound metabolic maintenance. An important by-product of increasing muscle mass is that the increased metabolic function will burn fat. The ability of lean muscle mass to cause an increase in the body's ability to burn fat is the reason why men, who generally have more muscle mass than women, tend to gain weight slower than women and lose weight faster than women.

We have established that muscle tissue can be replaced indefinitely. By the same token we know that metabolism can be affected indefinitely by the maintenance of adequate lean muscle mass, regardless of age. In the study at Tufts University mentioned earlier, a group of men and women engaged in strength training three days per week with impressive achievements in strength improvement. Their metabolic rate improved at about the same pace. On average, they increased their metabolisms by 15 percent, leading them to burn 200 to 300 extra calories every day over their previous rate.

A dietary note: Eating a high-carbohydrate, high-protein meal within half an hour after finishing a workout raises insulin levels, increases amino acid absorption into muscle, and speeds up the recovery process. The carbohydrates cause a spike in blood sugar that stimulates the pancreas to release insulin. Insulin drives the protein building blocks (amino acids) in the meal into muscle cells to hasten recovery from intense workouts. Muscles are extraordinarily sensitive to insulin during exercise and for up to a half hour after finishing exercise, so the fastest way to recover is to eat protein- and carbohydrate-rich foods shortly after you finish.

MUSCLES—A CRITICAL DEFENSE AGAINST DISEASE AND INJURY

Attending to your muscles is an investment that will yield dividends year after year. An additional payoff is the way that your musculature can ward off crippling injury and provide significant defense against a broad spectrum of diseases.

Osteoporosis

Loss of bone density, particularly in older women, has been a major factor in health issues. Hip fractures are the most serious and frequent complication of osteoporosis. In the United States there are close to half a million cases of hip fracture annually among people over 65. Most of these injuries are the result of falls, the majority of which would likely not occur if the individuals had maintained adequate muscle strength. About one in five hip fracture victims dies within a year of the accident. A quarter of those who had previously lived independently had to be confined to nursing homes after the accident.

A study that sought to understand the age-related decline in loss of bone mineral density examined the relative importance of muscle strength, physical fitness, and body mass index (BMI) in addition to age in the determination of femoral bone density in 73 healthy female volunteers ranging in age from 20 to 75. Muscle strength turned out to be the dominant factor correlated with bone density. General fitness was also associated with increasing bone density. However, age as an independent factor was not! Age was a predictor of osteoporosis only to the extent that age effects were exacerbated by deficiencies in muscle strength, physical fitness, or weight.

Cancer

Lean muscle mass may give even obese people an advantage in battling cancer, as shown by a study conducted at the University of Alberta. The study indicated that the body composition of cancer patients plays a role in survival rates, activity levels during the illness, and to some extent the reaction to chemotherapy treatment.

CAT scans of 250 obese cancer patients were viewed in the study to determine the amount of lean muscle mass. Those patients exhibiting sarcopenic obesity—a depletion of lean muscle mass associated with being severely overweight—had higher mortality rates than those patients with more normal muscle mass. They also tended to be bedridden much more, and have more loss of physical function.

The findings underscore the growing realization that body composition has to be taken into consideration when assessing patients in general. Lean muscle mass should be a consideration in how patients react to chemotherapy, drug dosages, and therapeutic strategies.

Psychological well-being

There are the all-important intangibles. Aging, we like to say, is a self-fulfilling prophecy. The attitudinal value of increasing strength at a time when we've been conditioned to expect decline is inestimable.

Numerous studies suggest that women who engage in strength training benefit from improved self-esteem. Female athletes consistently appear to be able to balance strength and femininity; according to one survey, 94 percent of the participants reported that strength training or athletic involvement did not incline them to feel less feminine.

Strength training also is widely credited with giving women a sense of personal power, especially among women who have suffered prior forms of abuse. Post-menopausal women can benefit from the sense of empowerment that new physical strength endows, as well as ward off the twin nemeses of frailty and osteoporosis.

The value of added strength and visible muscle to aging men goes almost without saying. It is a reaffirmation of cultural expectations of healthy masculinity and a symbolic refutation of decline as well as an eminently practicable one. Gaining strength is accompanied by increasing energy. It is a positive feedback cycle that makes additional health strategies appear more desirable as well as accessible.

Regardless of gender, the psychological value of *feeling strong* can be a priceless gift. To go through one's days not having to feel physically vulnerable, to carry the empowerment of knowing that you can simply deal with many of the physical challenges that you are likely to encounter, is enormously fulfilling and a great psychological boost.

A COMMITMENT TO STRENGTH

A PERSONAL PERSPECTIVE

by Randall Stickrod

As a child, one of my dominating memories was the sense of being a skinny, undersized kid with glasses, a bookworm pacifist growing up in the midst of tough rural kids, living in constant dread of being bullied. The notion of physical strength as a means toward carving out a secure niche for myself was surely a factor in my self-awareness of fitness and strength and physical capability from a tender age.

I began lifting weights (as well as doing hard physical labor) in my teens, and it developed into a kind of addiction. By the time I graduated from high school, I was clearly no longer that skinny, undersized kid who feared bullies. Growing up in the West had also given me a passion for the outdoors, for cherishing an intimate relationship with mountain and stream, and I have always relished treks into the wilderness, climbing and swimming and being able to embrace the physical world with zeal and confidence. The idea of building my strength seemed the perfect way to prepare myself for many of life's eventualities, both opportunities (physical adventure) and adversities (being able to respond effectively in life-threatening situations). And so it has proved to be.

As Dr. Bortz's own research has shown, we do decline naturally with age in most respects, and strength is no exception to that rule. Nevertheless, I have found that, even in my sixties now, I can do everything I did 20, 30, even 40 years ago. Today I am as strong as I ever was, a fact I attribute to two things, consistency and attitude. Consistency means always making resistance training a priority, no matter what else is going on. It means finding a way to get in that workout, no matter what. Thirty to 40 minutes every other day is a minimum baseline, and how hard can that be? Think of all the choices we make during a typical day of how to spend the next hour or two. What TV program might we live without? What lunch period might be put to better use in a gym? What trip to the store might also include a stop at the gym?

Attitude means a stubborn refusal to concede the upper hand to Mother Nature. I have gone to every workout these many years never once expecting to start doing less than I did in the previous workout. And now it is like a self-fulfilling prophecy, maintaining the same (or better!) level of strength that I had at 20.

Random observations:

- Somewhere in my thirties I decided that my fitness was a top priority and required real commitment. I never looked back. It was the easiest commitment I ever made.
- For many years I was traveling constantly and learned to be resourceful. I used to pack a long piece of surgical tubing for little workouts in a hotel room. It's amazing how much I could do with that by looping it around a door handle, for instance.
- Many years living in San Francisco, where there always seems to be construction scaffolding in front of buildings, led to a new rule— *never pass up a pull-up*. If I walked by the scaffolding, I'd always stop, get a handhold as high as I could, and do a few quick pull-ups, one of the best exercises ever.
- This may sound like heresy, but I get bored to death in gyms and have learned to make my workouts as quick as possible, rarely more

than 30 to 40 minutes, often less. The trick is to work quickly and intensively. Make your body work for it. Find your natural limits and work as close to them as you can without hurting yourself. When working with weights, find a weight that you can do ten repetitions with, but where the last couple takes a noticeable effort. Push yourself a little. You'll be pleasantly surprised to find out how well your body will respond to it, a firsthand lesson in phenotypic plasticity.

- When you get a routine down, vary it occasionally. Try a machine you've never tried before. Check out what other people are doing. Always be ready to learn something new. Surprise your body occasionally.

- When you least feel like working out often turns out to be the best time for it. The easiest thing in the world is to think of reasons not to work out. You're tired. You don't feel so good. You think you have a cold coming on. There are reasons galore. But once you decide to go, and do it, you always feel better. You are always glad you went. It is the great unacknowledged rule of working out—that no matter how you felt going in, you *always* feel glad you did it afterward. How many other things in life can make that same claim?

- And last, maybe the most important advice of all: Never be self-conscious. Never feel that it's a competition. Nobody else really cares what you're doing. The only person you are ever competing with is yourself. Be proud of yourself for getting to the gym and committing to a workout, even if you feel awkward and self-conscious about the way you look or the weight you're using. Nobody else cares, honestly!

CHAPTER 6

ENGAGEMENT:
THE NECESSITY OF
BEING NECESSARY

The probability of living to 100 and retaining your self-efficacy all the while is astonishingly good, as we have seen, if you embrace a life of movement. That is, if you systematically maintain your aerobic fitness and consciously strive to maintain sufficient lean muscle mass. The evidence is almost overwhelming. And yet we know, as sentient beings, that there is more to living than merely managing our metabolic needs.

There is an intangible factor that defies quantification but is a crucial part of who we are and how we live. Mme. Calment, who lived to 122 years, famously declared that she had "a great passion for living."

Without reasons to live, one might ask, why bother? The character of our will to live is one of the things that distinguishes us as unique beings, a hallmark of our individuality.

A variety of studies of centenarians has concluded that, aside from physical health, the intangible characteristics that stand out the most are optimism, hope, the ability to cope with loss, and engagement. Engagement is the expression of purpose. It is in our nature to seek purpose in our existence. We feel that engagement underlies all the other intangible factors; it allows us to find joy in living as long as possible.

We learn much from witnessing the absence of engagement. At one extreme, we know that sensory deprivation is lethal. The stimulation of ordinary daily experience is essential to our equilibrium. People who live in isolation rarely thrive. As we go through life, each of us has a "social convoy" of friends, family, and associates that accompanies us. In later years, many simply allow that convoy to vanish by attrition, taking with it a good part of the energy milieu that supports us. In studies of the social, emotional, and cognitive processes that accompany aging, Dr. Laura Carstensen of Stanford University has repeatedly found that once someone begins to consciously anticipate death, they tend to disengage.

Engagement comes in many flavors. Essentially it means a motivated involvement with factors outside oneself. It can be a spouse or mate. It can be family. It can be friends or community involvement.

More often in present times it is work or career. Sometimes it is a creative pursuit. Occasionally it is a combination of these.

Every centenarian has a story. There are often great variations in lifestyle, in diet, in the kinds of activities each engaged in, not to mention their socioeconomic circumstances. But the one thing that virtually all have had is a clear and often compelling sense of engagement. Therein lies not just a central part of the practical longevity formula, but a richness of human experience that is the foundation of our humanity.

Nearly all centenarians have many meaningful interpersonal relationships. They are almost never loners, and examples abound. For instance, one of the subjects of the New England Centenarian Study, William Cohen, 101 at last report, viewed independence as important to his longevity, but realized that a close family was just as important. "The goal when you're older is to keep family close," he said, "to be independent, but to have them to help. As you get older, you need people, not dollars and cents." It helps to have a capacity for social receptiveness. A Japanese study observed the lives of 70 cognitively intact Japanese centenarians aged 100 to 106 years alongside a larger group of elderly people aged 60 to 84 years, all residents of Tokyo. A survey was performed to assess five major personality traits: neuroticism, extraversion, openness, agreeableness, and conscientiousness. The results showed greater openness in both male and female centenarians, as well as higher conscientiousness and extraversion in female centenarians, when compared to those in the younger group. These results suggest that high scores in conscientiousness, extraversion, and openness are associated with longevity. Stated more simply, an outgoing personality creates more opportunity for social engagement and an enriched psychological environment. It is further thought that these personality traits contribute to longevity through health-related behavior, stress reduction, and adaptation to the challenges of extreme old age.

There is a well-known correlation between social isolation and suicide as well as sociopathic behaviors. The kind of despair that usually leads one to no longer value living is usually bred in isolation; narrowing one's focus shuts out the constructive dynamics of interaction with others. We are social creatures by nature, and draw life-giving energy from our interactions with other people. This can be thought of as analogous to the energy requirements of our cells, where cellular function is driven by energy exchanges with the cellular environment. Energy is life.

Our longevity benchmark, Mme. Calment, provides a fantastic example of someone who actively and eagerly participated in this social energy exchange. She was exceedingly social and claimed to have a good appetite for food and everything else. She enjoyed port wine and chocolates (and an occasional cigarette) along with her social involvements. She rode a bicycle at 100, but, most telling, claimed that "I never get bored." Her life was a model of energy interchange. She was fully engaged.

Centenarian case studies invariably focus on the engagement dimension, either socially (including family) or in terms of work, including creative engagement. The artist known as Grandma Moses took up painting rural landscapes for her own pleasure in her late seventies, though she had no prior training. She was still painting at 100, nearly every day, and produced at least 25 original works after her 100th birthday, demonstrating the power of creative engagement. The painter Pablo Picasso was an exemplar of creative engagement through the full cycle of his life; perhaps if he had taken a little better care of himself physically, he may well have continued beyond his mere 92 years.

George Dawson, the grandson of a slave, worked all his life and at the age of 98 decided that he was tired of writing his name with an X, so he learned to read and write. At 102 he co-wrote the story of his life, *Life Is So Good,* and earned his GED at age 103.

Fred Sheill runs a ten-acre lily nursery in Au Gres, Michigan, at 100, continuing a passion for small-scale agriculture that began at age 12. With the help of a gaggle of tame geese that eat insects and weeds, he continues to work full days, growing some 500,000 daylilies a year. A typical day involves driving a tractor to compost his crops, spending time with customers, and driving around distributing brochures advertising his flowers. He claims to "always be making plans for next year."

Attorney Jack Borden, 101, of Weatherford, Texas, continues to practice law, specializing in real estate and wills, sometimes finding himself working with a fifth generation of clients. At 101 he puts in a 40-hour-long workweek. Coming to work and being with people "keeps me alive," he has said. "I'll keep working and someday they'll find me here with my head on the desk."

Engagement is strongly associated with functional independence, or self-efficacy. The landmark New England Centenarian Study, which began in 1994 and is an expanding, ongoing, comprehensive study of centenarian case histories, brought special attention to self-efficacy and successful independent lifestyles of the elderly. It found that 90 percent of the centenarians studied were functionally independent over the vast majority of their lives up until the age of 92, on average, and 75 percent were still fully independent at 95. That independence was strongly correlated with strong social or family connections. Social contacts were just far enough away that the subject lived independently, but near enough to be closely bonded and part of a natural support system.

Dr. Will Miles Clark, 105, of Tucson, Arizona, is a retired dentist whose wife, Lois, is also a centenarian. At 105 he was still driving his Toyota Sienna, playing golf regularly, and reading compulsively, claiming never to be without a book. Lois plays bridge, a pastime that is increasingly linked with successful aging. Dr. Clark got his first computer in 2009, took a few lessons, and learned to book their vacation getaways online.

Elsa Hoffmann, 102, of Hillsboro Beach, Florida, lives a social life that people of any age might envy. She plays bridge and gin, regularly goes out for dinner and drinks, and is known in her social circle as an incurable optimist. Her "secret" is that she loves to "make people happy" and that "I live every day grateful that I'm here and that I can be useful." She has always played golf and after knee surgery at 86 came back to play what she claims was the best golf game of her life. She has always been conscious of her diet, with an emphasis on fruit and very little fried food. And most tellingly, she feels that she is nearly as active at 102 as she ever was.

A long-term study of nearly 4,000 Japanese American men living in Honolulu, Hawaii, looked for a connection between social engagement and dementia as the subjects aged. But first the researchers asked what, exactly, do we mean by social engagement, and how do we measure it? They chose five measures: marital status, living arrangement (alone or with others), participation in group activities (community, social, or political groups), participation in social events with others (movies, dancing, etc.), and the existence of a confidante relationship or close personal friend. A system of scoring was established, and each subject earned a total score from these five factors. How these levels of engagement changed over time was then analyzed.

Several facts stood out. First, men who had high scores throughout the period had the least occurrence of dementia, an unequivocal correlation. Having a pattern of strong social bonds early in life and then maintaining that pattern into later life is an excellent way to guard against dementia in all its usual forms. Second, those whose level of social engagement declined from midlife to late life had the highest risk of dementia. The greater the decline, the greater the probability of onset of dementia.

Another observation from the study was that lower levels of midlife engagement were typically found in participants with lower levels of education. It has been said, somewhat offhandedly, that smart people live longer. It may be more accurate to say that better-educated people live longer because they have an ability to make better lifestyle choices and perhaps more reasons to form varieties of social bonds that carry over into later life.

We can only partially verify why this is, but the data is convincing. There are several reasons why social engagement could reduce the risk of dementia. In studies with animals (the kind where testing on humans directly is simply not possible), environmental inputs that are both complex and richly diverse prevent cognitive decline and actually encourage neurogenesis (the creation of new neuronal cells in the brain). It is thought that social and physical activity may increase a person's ability to overcome brain pathologies because enhanced synaptic activity promotes more efficient brain recovery and repair.

It is also believed that social experiences may reduce the risk of dementia by reducing both stress and cardiovascular disease risk factors that are also associated with brain diseases. Hormones, including corticosteroids, are affected by the stress reduction associated with social engagement, and these hormones have wide-ranging benefits, including an improved immune response, better carbohydrate metabolism, and inflammation control.

A Harvard research group was interested in knowing why some people with chronic diseases have the ability to live into their eighties or nineties, when others with similar health profiles succumb decades earlier. In findings published in August 1999 in the *British Medical Journal*, they came up with a surprising answer.

In their study of nearly 3,000 people 65 and older who were followed for a period of 13 years, the researchers tracked participation in 14 activities, which included everything from swimming and brisk walking to shopping, doing volunteer work, and regular group social activities like playing cards. They found that people who spent regular time in social activities—as simple as volunteering, running errands, or getting together with friends—fared just as well as those who spent the equivalent time exercising. Social engagement was the single strongest factor in the longevity of this group, stronger than exercise, blood pressure, cholesterol, and other standard health metrics.

In another study, a team from the University of Michigan interviewed and examined 2,754 adults over a period of 9 to 12 years. Their results, published in the *American Journal of Epidemiology*, showed that men who reported more social relationships—going to movies, church meetings, classes, or trips with friends or relatives, for example—were significantly less likely to die during the study period. Socially active women also benefited, although not quite as dramatically, probably because the women were already on track to live longer than the men, since women typically have longer life spans than men under all circumstances.

> *People who spent regular time in social activities—as simple as volunteering, running errands, or getting together with friends—fare just as well as those who spent the equivalent time exercising.*

Marriage, too, turns out to have important health benefits. Researchers at Bordeaux University in France reported that among 2,800 volunteers followed over a five-year period, married people were one-third less likely than the never-married to develop Alzheimer's disease.

There are an abundance of reasons why your ties to friends, family, and loved ones may keep you healthy. A spouse can care for you when you get sick, for instance, which may mean a faster recovery from serious illnesses. People with the support of friends or spouses typically feel a greater sense of self-esteem and so take better care of themselves by adopting a healthy lifestyle. A strong social network may also help reduce stress, and there's ample evidence that psychological well-being can have a strong positive effect on physical health.

A strong and positive attitude boosts the immune system, which wards off disease. People who are lonely or socially isolated show signs of suppressed immunity, according to Ohio State University immunologist Ronald Glaser, who, along with his wife, Janice Kiecolt-Glaser, pioneered the study of how mental states affect the immune system. In a 1984 study, they found that patients who scored above the median level on loneliness tests, meaning they were more lonely than the average person, had significantly fewer active natural killer cells—lymphocyte cells that attack intruders, including tumors and viruses.

The importance of a social dimension to successful aging cannot be overstated. There is a growing sense among gerontologists that, as a society, we should be finding more ways for older people to stay involved and active. It is becoming clear that exercise therapies are coming up short if there is not a social dimension as well.

Physical fitness is critical, as we have shown in previous chapters, but social engagement is probably equally critical to longevity. In the geriatrics profession now, there are increasing advisories for older people to find something they really like doing that involves other people, from taking walks together to playing cards together to attending events together.

But these advisories, well intentioned as they are, don't adequately portray a complete or fully informed picture. While there is undeniable merit in urging people to change their patterns and somewhat artificially seek out engagement opportunities, the best case is one in which engagement springs naturally from one's life interests. When one is following a passionate interest in midlife and simply carries it forward into later life, the motive force is internally generated and fueled by an organic passion. It's why many artists have long, productive lives, driven as they are by the need (and the satisfaction) associated with the creative process.

In Gloucester in the United Kingdom, Ralph Hoare is known as the 101-year-old golfer to some and the 101-year-old gardener to others. He also plays the piano seriously and has an enviable circle of friends. The first three activities are passions; the social dimension is a natural complement. His longevity surprises no one who knows him.

We call it *the necessity of being necessary.* When there is internal purpose, when one is driven by a passionate desire or buoyed up by the force of one's relationships, then one has the best of all possible worlds, and a kind of continuity of forces is at work that conspires to keep one young, strong, and at the top of one's game.

An exemplary model is the life of Albert H. Gordon, long-time head of investment bank Kidder Peabody. Gordon died in mid-2009 at the age of 107. He was known not just for his legendary success in business (masterminding Kidder Peabody's rise from insolvency after the crash of 1929 to success as the second-largest investment bank at its prime), but for the humanness of his management style and the quality of his relationships. He was deeply engaged in business, making client calls well into his nineties, and worked four days a week at 105. He was vitally active with his extensive non-business interests until the end. It should also be noted that he was legendary for his physical fitness as well, which he felt was central to his longevity. Twice he was the oldest participant in the London marathon. When traveling, he was known to occasionally walk from the airport to his hotel.

A life of engagement is the perfect expression of life as a self-fulfilling prophecy. We who live long and healthy will do so because we expect to.

CHAPTER 7

SEX AND THE LIFE FORCE

It seems a bit odd that, nearly 40 years after Alex Comfort's huge best-seller, *The Joy of Sex,* we are a culture still snarled up in conflicting and confusing attitudes about sex and the role of sexuality in our lives. When it comes to aging and the elderly, the issue of sex becomes even more muddled, often bordering on the taboo. It's as if society has drawn an age boundary around sex, making it permissible only in a range between the late teens and somewhere in late middle age. Though it's easy enough to find professional advice asserting the right to sexuality among the elderly as well as the revelation that people of very advanced years are still having sex (horrors!), many are still generally uncomfortable with the notion as a rule.

It is no secret that older people continue to have sex. As the baby boomer generation enters their fifties and sixties, they seem unlikely to

give up sex simply because they are "of a certain age." But sex among
the aging is not a new phenomenon. There are studies galore to confirm
this, though most show a predictable tapering off with increasing age.
One found that around 70 percent of men were sexually active at 68,
but that by 78, just ten years later, that percentage had dropped to 25
percent. A more generous survey polling healthy 80- to 102-year-olds
found that 63 percent of men and 30 percent of women were still having sexual intercourse. The disparity between men and women is surely
exacerbated by the fact that as the years roll up, men die sooner than
women as a rule, and by the age of 80, there are only 39 men for every
100 women. Regardless, no matter which survey one chooses to look
at, the fact is that sexual desire, sexual activity, and concerns with sex go
on indefinitely.

And why shouldn't they? Sex is at the very root of our life force, intrinsic to the very spark and pulse of life. It contains the essence of who
we are as living organisms, and the sex act is a perfect affirmation of life
itself.

Sexuality is, to be sure, an appropriately complex issue. It invokes
the whole experience of self, including relationships with others, feelings about oneself, and the functioning of the body. Nothing is so
powerful an integrating mechanism between mind and body as sex.
How could sex *not* be an important variable in our personal health
equation?

So let's start with the assumption that sex is normal, healthy, and natural. But will it *make* you healthier? Will it help you live longer—is it on the critical path to 100? It is fairly well known that being in good health is linked to good sex. The question becomes, in a chicken-or-egg sort of way, is the converse true? Does sex lead to better health and a longer life?

A handful of studies make unequivocal claims for the health and longevity benefits of a robust sex life. The first serious systematic investigation of this was a 1997 study of Welsh men. It found that men who claimed two or more orgasms per week at the time of the study had less than half the risk of dying from various causes over ten years of follow-up than those with a lower frequency of orgasm.

> *A handful of studies make unequivocal claims for the health and longevity benefits of a robust sex life. The first serious systematic investigation of this was a 1997 study of Welsh men. It found that men who claimed two or more orgasms per week at the time of the study had less than half the risk of dying from various causes over ten years of follow-up than those with a lower frequency of orgasm.*

The study results strongly pointed to a dose-response relationship between frequency of orgasm and mortality. That is, the more orgasms you have, the longer you live. By extension of these results, one could infer that daily sex should add at least eight years to a man's life span.

The researchers noted rather dryly that "If these findings are replicated, there are implications for health promotion programs."

At Duke University, a longevity study that began in the 1950s found that the frequency of sexual intercourse (for men) and the enjoyment of sex (for women) were clearly linked to longevity. Other studies have found that sexual *dis*satisfaction could be a predictor of the onset of cardiovascular disease. One compared 100 women with heart disease (acute myocardial infarction) with a control group and found lack of sexual response and dissatisfaction with their sex life among 65 percent of the coronary patients, but only 24 percent of the control group. Though in all this research correlations were found between the frequency or enjoyment of sex and longevity or other outcomes, these studies do not fully answer the "chicken or egg" question. But the consistent association of sexual activity and enjoyment with health and longevity is indisputable.

Another long-term study in Scotland, covering people between the ages of 30 and 101, concluded that, at the very least, sex helps you look younger. Subjects with active sex lives were judged to appear four to seven years younger than they actually were. Researchers attributed this to the therapeutic effects of significant stress reduction, improved sleep, and overall contentment that comes from regular sex. Other researchers have added the benefits of intimacy and improved personal relationships as factors deriving from sex that lead to better health and increased longevity. Sex and health have been described as part of a "virtuous cycle"; they reinforce each other.

MEN'S SEXUAL HEALTH

As a man ages, his testosterone levels decrease. Typically this decrease in testosterone begins around the age of 40 and declines quite slowly, tending to stabilize around age 60. A reduction in testosterone can lead to less muscle mass and strength, less red blood cell production, decreasing bone density, increasing fat, and, of course, a decreasing sex drive. Maintaining adequate levels of testosterone to sustain a healthy libido as well as stable muscle mass is an important strategy for maintaining the vitality that will help one get to 100 fit and functional.

Synthetic testosterone has been produced and is available for replacement therapies, though not without cautionary advisories. Testosterone replacement therapy is becoming increasingly popular among aging men as a quick fix to restore youthfulness. We are all familiar with the dark side of this treatment, evidenced most recently in the steroid scandals in professional sports. The problems with testosterone supplements are many and the subject of ongoing controversies. The possibility of sterility, hair loss, and heart enlargement, and even the potential of accelerating prostate cancer, to name a few of the possible side effects, make a steep price to pay for the superficial benefits that the supplements yield.

Fortunately, most men have a built-in testosterone-producing engine, and that is exercise. But not all forms of exercise. The duration, intensity, and frequency of exercise will determine the circulating levels of testosterone. Testosterone levels increase most with short, intense bursts of activity, like weight training or sprinting, while levels decrease with prolonged activity, especially that of frequent endurance training. During endurance training, testosterone is needed to maintain muscle, but frequent extended training doesn't allow for repair and recovery of testosterone, leading to possible tissue damage in the stressed muscles.

Studies show that testosterone levels will elevate with exercise for about 45 to 60 minutes. After this amount of time, cortisol—the "stress hormone"—levels begin to increase and testosterone levels tend to decline. This decrease has been detected for up to six days following exercise.

Men who exercise are less likely to experience sexual dysfunction as they get older. Analyzing data from surveys of nearly 32,000 men ages 53 to 90, researchers concluded that men who were the most physically active were least likely to become impotent. According to Eric B. Rimm, an associate professor at the Harvard School of Public Health, men who ran at least three hours per week appeared to have the sexual functioning of men two to five years younger. But even moderate activity proved beneficial: Men who briskly walked for 30 minutes, most days of the week, had a 15 to 20 percent reduction in the risk of erectile dysfunction.

What this suggests is a win-win proposition for men who engage in a balanced exercise program of cardiovascular (aerobic) and weight-training (anaerobic) exercise, the latter to maintain testosterone levels and the former to keep key arteries healthy. Aerobic exercise improves the function of the small arteries that control erections, for the same reason that exercise is good for the heart. Enlarged arteries as the result of consistent exercise—phenotypic plasticity at work—facilitate optimum blood flow to the organ. And while many men may act indifferently about their heart health, they may be more motivated to do something about the health of their sex lives. With fewer than 25 percent of Americans getting enough exercise, it is not surprising that sexual dysfunction has crept so prominently into the modern vocabulary, particularly among older men. In a related vein, some doctors believe that impotence could be considered an early warning sign of heart trouble, another good reason to pay heed to these vital processes.

Much has been made of the discovery of erectile dysfunction drugs. While pharmaceutical solutions are always less preferable than more natural and broadly health-inducing forms of remediation, drugs such as Viagra and Cialis appear to have no serious side effects and are commendable for extending the sex lives of many who might otherwise find themselves unable to participate. It should be noted, however, that context is important. The health-enhancing and life-extending benefits of sex are not a function of merely getting an erection and an ejaculation. Sex facilitates emotional bonding, relationship dynamics, and attitudinal factors consistent with the assertion of good health and the celebration of life.

Prostate cancer, the specter overshadowing modern male health, is not to be taken lightly. Though detection and treatment strategies continue to improve, shrinking mortality rates, prostate cancer's threat to an active sex life is real and foreboding. But as we learned in Chapter 4, prostate health can be significantly bolstered by consistent aerobic exercise. As a preventive strategy, exercise is the one defensive action that is accessible to everyone, every day, and that has a known measure of proven effectiveness.

WOMEN'S SEXUAL HEALTH

The convergence of aging and sex presents a somewhat different and more complex lineup of issues for women than for men. Some involve physiological changes unique to women (for example, post-menopausal hormone changes, vaginal dryness), but aside from those, the issues of health benefits and longevity factors bear little difference from those presented to men.

As women age, many may experience dwindling interest in sex, but that doesn't mean women aren't sexually active or have lost all desire. A recent study on "Sexual Function and Aging in Racially and Ethnically Diverse Women" at the University of California at San Francisco examined the sexual behaviors of nearly 2,000 women, aged 45 to 80 years old. Of these, 43 percent reported at least moderate sexual desire, and 60 percent had been sexually active in the previous three months. Half of all sexually active participants described their overall sexual satisfaction as moderate to high. More than one-quarter of women aged 65 years or older remained moderately or highly interested in sex, and more than one-third of women in this age group had been sexually active in the past three months.

Among sexually inactive women in the entire group, the most common reason was related to partner problems, which accounted for 70 percent of the responses. These included lack of a partner (36 percent), physical problems of a partner (23 percent), and lack of interest by a partner (11 percent).

Despite the fact that the prevalence of sexual activity did decrease with increasing age, overall, 37 percent of the women who were 65 and older were sexually active in the past three months, and about that percentage were moderately or highly interested in sex.

Women who are happy with their sex lives have higher well-being scores and more vitality than women who are sexually dissatisfied, according to an Australian research effort from Monash University led by Dr. Sonia Davison. They tracked a group of women who reported having sex at least twice a month, in order to discover links between sexual satisfaction and overall well-being, and additionally to see if post-menopausal women registered significantly different results than younger women.

They found that women who were sexually dissatisfied had lower well-being and lower vitality scores. The researchers noted that these findings underscore the importance of directly addressing sexual satisfaction as an essential part of women's health, because women may be uncomfortable bringing up these issues with their doctor. More than 90 percent of the women in the study said their sexual activity involved a partner, and that sexual activity was initiated by the partner at least 50 percent of the time. This means that the sexual activity of the study participants may have been affected by partner presence/absence, partner health, and sexual function—factors that weren't addressed in the study, the researchers noted.

This dimension tends to be one significant differentiation between the way women and men must be interpreted in these investigations. The fact that women who self-identified as being dissatisfied maintained the level of sexual activity reported most likely represents established behavior and partner expectation. It also reinforces the fact that frequency of sexual activity in women cannot be employed by itself as a reliable indicator of sexual well-being.

By far the most common sexual problem that women report in their post-reproductive years is dyspareunia—pain or discomfort during or after intercourse or other penetration of the vagina. After menopause, reduced levels of the hormones estrogen and progesterone tend to result in less natural lubrication and more discomfort, or even painful sex.

There are remedies, however. Likely the best, and most obvious, is simply regular sex. Many women and sex therapists confirm the essential truth of the "use it or lose it" dictum. Regular sex, including masturbation, definitely helps keep vaginal glands active and tissues supple and moist. Extended sex play before penetration is always helpful even if discomfort isn't severe. Liberal use of a water-soluble lubricant is often enough to make intercourse more comfortable.

Low libido, or a loss of sexual arousal in women, can be an indicator of other underlying conditions. High cholesterol, for instance, isn't just bad for the heart—it could also make it harder for women to become sexually aroused. That might mean that cholesterol-lowering drugs like statins would help to treat so-called female sexual dysfunction (FSD).

Hyperlipidemia, or raised levels of cholesterol and other fats in the blood, is associated with erectile dysfunction in men, because the buildup of fats in blood vessel walls can reduce blood flow to erectile tissue. Since some aspects of female sexual arousal also rely on increased blood flow to the genitals, a research group at the Second University of Naples

in Italy studied sexual function in premenopausal women, both with
and without hyperlipidemia.

Women with hyperlipidemia reported significantly lower arousal,
orgasm, lubrication, and sexual satisfaction scores than women with
normal blood lipid profiles. And 32 percent of the women with abnor-
mal profiles scored low enough on a scale of female sexual function to
be diagnosed with FSD, compared with 9 percent of women without
normal levels. Women's sexual desire was not affected by hyperlipidemia, however.

In a separate paper, Annamaria Veronelli at the University of Milan,
Italy, and her colleagues found that female sexual dysfunction was also
associated with diabetes, obesity, and an underactive thyroid gland.
These factors also apply to men, of course.

In fact, these two studies point to strong connections between
women's sexual arousal and organic diseases that parallel the way that
men's sexual problems arise. This parallelism has barely been recognized
in the current research, and is rarely even considered in women.

A fairly new term, hypoactive sexual desire disorder (HSDD), has
begun appearing in the medical literature on the heels of a burst of new
studies and, not coincidentally, an equivalent burst of interest from
pharmaceutical companies looking to cash in on "the next Viagra." Discussions of HSDD break out into two separate categories: issues of
arousal and issues of desire. Arousal issues focus on physiological re-

sponse, such as lubrication and orgasm, whereas the desire focus is on the psychological factors of lessened interest in sex. All of this will likely lead to a new wave of pharmaceutical remedies such as the drug fil-banserin, which has shown promise in clinical trials, though all its pathways and consequences have yet to be fully explicated.

It should be noted that the array of herbal products promising libido-lifting effects has never stood up to scientific studies. Sex is one area where male-female symmetries tend to break down, not just physiologically but culturally as well. We inhabit a cultural milieu that too often promotes shame and ignorance about women's sexuality while wildly inflating their expectations for sex. This underscores the importance of recognizing that the power of our sexuality requires context—psychological comfort, absence of stress, supportive relationships, physical well-being—in other words, the full array of health factors that support a long life.

AN ASIDE—STRATEGIES
FOR STAYING SEXUAL

Many of us seem to feel that sex is something that is supposed to happen without a great deal of thought or consideration, as if it were like hunger, say, or an itch to be scratched. That kind of attitude deprives us of the full possibilities of sex as a way of enhancing life, much as if one regards food as merely fuel and goes through life without appreciating the deep pleasures of gastronomy.

There are a variety of self-help solutions available to women to enhance their interest in, and enjoyment during, sex. Heterosexual women and lesbians clearly have the same problems, but lesbians may find it easier to negotiate solutions because their partners may have similar issues. If intercourse is painful or male partners don't get erections readily, consider taking the focus off of intercourse and discover the pleasures of "outercourse," which includes any sexual activity except penis-in-vagina sex. The principle is to shift the goal of sexual activity from orgasm to pleasure. One should not have to "work" toward orgasm. It has been said that sex should begin with willingness and end with pleasure, with or without orgasm along the way. Since it's the brain, and not the genitals, that's our chief sex organ, a little thoughtfulness can go a long way toward sexual enjoyment. Rewarding sex can be as simple as creative cuddling, sensual massages, sharing fantasies, genital touching, or indulging in erotica together. If there is genital response to these activities, with or without touching, it's still sex!

TOUCH—THE HIDDEN DIMENSION OF SEXUALITY

The full dimension of our sexual nature—our human nature—includes the psycho-physical effects of touch, and not just sex-specific contact.

The biochemical responses we generate at the cellular and glandular level that give us our sense of healthy well-being can be invoked by touch. Without feeling the requirement to draw on a lot of rigorous science, we feel we can simply state that touch is good, that it's beneficial to our overall health. We know from the previous chapter the essential role of engagement. It takes no great leap of logic to understand the connection between engagement and touch.

Touch is necessary for mammals to thrive, a fact well understood by pet owners and people involved in animal husbandry. Animals and babies deprived of physical touch are likely to be sickly and do not develop at normal rates. How touch impacts health is not entirely understood, but touch apparently works on several levels, and includes a direct hormonal link.

Researchers at the University of California, San Diego, School of Medicine have been studying the brain hormone that is released with touches and hugs, or when a mother and her newborn baby bond. They feel this hormone might help patients with schizophrenia, social anxiety, and a variety of other disorders.

Oxytocin is a brain chemical associated with pair bonding, including mother-infant and male-female bonds, increased paternal involvement with children, and monogamy in certain rodents. In humans, oxytocin is released during hugging and pleasant physical touch, and comes into play in the human sexual response cycle. It appears to change the brain signals related to social recognition via facial expressions, perhaps by changing the firing of the amygdala, the part of the brain that plays a primary role in the processing of important emotional stimuli. In this way, oxytocin in the brain may be a potent mediator of human social behavior.

That's why oxytocin is sometimes called the love hormone. The eyes may or may not be the "window to the soul," but they are a window to the emotional brain. We know that eye-to-eye communication—which is affected by oxytocin—is critical to intimate emotional communication for a wide range of emotions linked to interpersonal relations.

The benefits of touch roughly sort out in the following categories. Touch:

1. Facilitates weight gain in pre-term infants
2. Enhances attentiveness
3. Alleviates depressive symptoms
4. Ameliorates pain
5. Reduces stress hormone production
6. Improves immune function

BEING SEXY, FEELING SEXY

Our sexuality, our self-awareness as a sexual being, can be a self-fulfilling prophecy. If we have insecure, troubled, or conflicted feelings about sex or our own sexuality or sexual experiences, these feelings and attitudes can have a marked effect on our physical welfare. We have already seen the extent to which physical sex and our physical health are interconnected. What we think and what we then project are part of that same information loop. Negative feelings (or non-feelings) can launch a downward spiral of sexual negativity. Conversely, positive attitude, the embrace of one's sexuality, can ignite or keep lit the flames of a healthy and rewarding sex life.

Feeling sexy stimulates the production of various hormones and enhances the intangible ways we interact with other human beings. We all know this from our youth; extending the principle to our later years can literally be a life-giving strategy.

CHAPTER 8

THE HEALTHY

AGING BRAIN

The erosion of mental capacity with advancing age is something we've generally taken for granted, accepted as an inevitable *coup de grâce* by Mother Nature. It seems somehow a way of adding insult to injury after the physical debilitation that was usually associated with growing old. We have a tendency to regard mental acuity in the elderly as something exceptional—"Uncle Jack is pretty sharp—for an 80-year-old guy!" We make self-conscious jokes about "senior moments" to account for lapses in memory. And all of this is supported by commonly accepted lore that we lose brain cells with age.

Behind this lore is the fact that neuroscience has done little to dispel these notions until very recently. For decades it was commonly believed that all 100 billion of our brain cells existed at birth, that the adult human brain cannot grow new cells, and that memory works by rewiring old brain cells rather than by growing new brain cells to record new data. In other words, the loss of brain cells over time was considered irreversible.

Breakthrough experiments in the late 1990s showed us that the brain is dynamic and changes and grows throughout our lives. Scientists at the Salk Institute, a Swedish university, and then Princeton University, as reported in *The Scientist,* found they were able to replicate natural processes that produced new neurons. These new brain cells migrated up into the cortex and established synapses with older cells in the frontal lobes (where personality, planning, decision making, and working memory are located) and in the parietal lobes (where visual recognition memory exists). Shortly after, scientists at Cornell were able to observe a similar process in the hippocampus, which is associated with memory and spatial memory and is usually one of the first casualties of Alzheimer's disease. The creation of new brain cells (neurogenesis) had been observed in animals for many years but was thought to be unlikely in the higher regions of the human brain.

Neurogenesis is activated and controlled by compounds called neurotrophins, primarily brain-derived neurotrophic factor (BDNF), a protein that is encoded by the BDNF gene. BDNF functions to help support the survival of existing neurons and encourages the growth and differentiation of new neurons and synapses, which we can think of as neuronal plasticity. It is active in the cortex and hippocampus, where learning, memory, and analytical thinking predominate. If BDNF is the key to brain cell regeneration, what, then, must we do to maintain a high level of BDNF?

Exercise, particularly aerobic exercise, is the answer. A recent study at Columbia University put a group of subjects, ages 21 through 45, through an exercise workout program four times a week, one hour per day, and then conducted a variety of measurements at the 12-week mark. Not surprisingly, the subjects all become more fit, a fact confirmed by much higher VO_2 max scores. Then they were subjected to functional MRI scans of their brains, which measured not only the physical size and shape of the brain, but also the blood flow and electrical activity within the brain.

The MRI results were stunning. In parts of each subject's brain, the blood volume had nearly doubled after a mere 12 weeks on the exercise regimen. The hippocampus was the focal point. In addition to the various reasons brain cells can die or get injured, brain volume tends to shrink with age, a process that often starts in your thirties. The hippocampus is particularly vulnerable to shrinking. It is widely believed that the loss of neurons in the hippocampus, regardless of the reason, is the principal cause of the cognitive decline associated with typical aging. Dementia, including Alzheimer's, is invariably accompanied by a smaller hippocampus.

Researchers concluded that exercise can stop or slow down age-related shrinkage of the hippocampus and its attendant neurological deficiencies. Test subjects who achieved the highest VO_2 max scores also scored highest on memory testing at the end of the study.

The Columbia results have now been repeated in other studies. At the University of Illinois, a study group of elderly people (ages 60 to 79) who had been largely sedentary began a program of walking an hour a day, three times a week. After six months, MRI scans not only showed significant growth in several parts of the brain, but suggested that we have the ability to produce new blood vessels and to strengthen neural connections as well as create new brain cells. Another group with a similar profile participated in non-aerobic exercises, primarily stretching and "toning" exercises, and in addition, one other group of young adults didn't participate in any of the exercise programs but were used for comparison in the MRI scanning data. The non-aerobic group showed no changes in brain tissue at all. And the younger group that did no exercises also showed no changes. The case for aerobic exercise as the path to brain health seemed incontrovertible.

Simply providing more blood to the brain seems intuitively a good thing. More blood means more oxygen, but there is more than oxygen behind neurogenesis. It is instructive to look a bit deeper into what is actually happening that is keeping the brain in top form. There are a number of theories, all of which have credence. One credits exercise with helping to "push" a key protein through what is known as the blood-brain barrier. The insulin-like protein is a growth factor that is produced in greater amounts in response to aerobic exercise. Exercise also stimulates the brain to produce more serotonin, a mood-affecting hormone that is also associated with neuron growth. Low serotonin levels are often seen in cases of clinical depression. It has been suggested that Prozac, the immensely popular antidepressant, might just as well be replaced in many cases by an exercise prescription, since both take several weeks to begin having an effect, and often deliver the same results.

Improving brain capacity and function through exercise doesn't have to be exclusively for the benefit of older people. Several programs have been instituted for schoolchildren with remarkable results. In a 2007 trial, 259 Illinois third and fifth graders were put through a series of standard physical education routines and had their body mass measured. Then their physical results were measured against their math and reading scores on the Illinois Standards Achievement Test. The more physical tests they passed, the better they scored on the achievement test. The effects appeared regardless of gender or socioeconomic differences, supporting the conclusion that the fitness of a child's body and the fitness of the mind are tightly linked.

In another study published the same year, researchers found that children ages 7 to 11 who exercised for 40 minutes daily after school had greater academic improvement than same-aged kids who worked out for just 20 minutes. In other words, the larger the amount of exercise, the greater the payoff in academic achievement.

An ongoing program for high school students begun in 2005, also in Illinois, is systematically championing exercise for academic gains. In the pilot program, students participated for 30 minutes in aerobic drills, wearing heart monitors to ensure that their heart rate was in the target zone of 160–190 beats per minute. Then they joined other students, who had not exercised, in a special literacy class. The students who took PE prior to class showed one and a quarter year's improvement on the standardized reading test after just one semester, while the exercise-free students gained just nine-tenths of a year.

The same approach was then applied to math-troubled students, with part of the class taking the PE regimen before an introductory algebra class. The results were even more dramatic. Exercising students increased their math test scores by more than 20 percent, while the rest gained less than 4 percent. It was found that the time of day the students exercised didn't make a difference. What mattered was taking the academic class immediately following PE, or when the effects of maximum circulation in the brain were still significant.

If exercise is a key stimulant for brain cell regrowth, one might expect that obesity could be a negative factor. That seems to be the case, yet another health concern associated with excessive weight. A recent UCLA study of 94 people in their seventies found that obese people have 8 percent less brain tissue than normal-weight individuals. Their brains looked 16 years older than the brains of lean individuals, according to researchers. And it's not just obesity. Those classified as merely overweight showed 4 percent less brain tissue than their normal-weight peers, and their brains appeared to have aged prematurely by eight years.

Researchers felt these numbers represented "severe brain degeneration," as a result of the loss of tissue, and a serious depletion of cognitive reserves, greatly increasing the risk of dementia and a broad class of other diseases that affect the brain. Obese people had lost brain tissue in the frontal and temporal lobes, areas of the brain critical for planning and memory, as well as the areas designated for attention and executive functions, long-term memory, and movement, according to the research report. Overweight people were affected less severely, but still showed brain loss in the area of long-term memory. The study concluded that the most strenuous kind of exercise can save about the same amount of brain tissue that is lost in the obese.

MEMORY

The brain is the vault for our most precious resource, our accumulated experience. Experience ultimately represents a survival device, since it represents the knowledge we have gained—and continue to accrue—

over the course of our life. The physiology of memory is a thrilling narrative of discovery, of complex labyrinths and the constant emergence of new synaptic connections, joining together previously unconnected dendritic branches. Without active intervention, it is also a story of degradation and loss.

The importance of a high level of circulation and oxygenation within the brain, particularly the amygdala, which plays such a pivotal role in memory, is critical, as we have shown. In addition, there are a variety of memory-training strategies extant that can make a profound difference, often restoring name recall and computational skills in the elderly to levels not seen since they were in their twenties. This asserts the important adage, "It's not the cards you are dealt, but how you play the hand." Living 100 years would be a lesser achievement if it occurred without one's memory to accompany the journey.

ALZHEIMER'S DISEASE

A report from the Alzheimer's Association predicts that ten million baby boomers will develop the disease in the United States, a figure that translates to about one out of every eight. Dr. Ronald Petersen, director of the Alzheimer's Research Center at the Mayo Clinic, has gone on the record stating that "Regular physical exercise is probably the best means we have of preventing Alzheimer's disease today, better than medications, better than intellectual activity, better than supplements and diet." This is a refrain being heard from an increasing number of dementia researchers, that to fight against these diseases we must focus on heart fitness.

Columbia University Medical Center in New York found that the risk of Alzheimer's was reduced by a third in volunteers who were physically active. Those who combined a fitness regimen with a healthy diet strategy with an emphasis on fruits and vegetables lowered their risk by a massive 60 percent.

These findings are all relatively recent and have received disproportionately less public attention than they deserve. That is most likely accounted for by the fact that the vast majority of attention is focused on pharmaceutical efforts. Spending on Alzheimer's drugs in 2010 is estimated to be in excess of $6 billion, an enormous market. To date, pharmaceutical-based therapies have been only modestly successful at best, never really curing the patient, but simply ameliorating some of the effects of the disease or slowing its progress. This all seems remarkable considering that the most effective preventive strategy as well as therapeutic approach is accessible to all and costs nothing.

After cardiovascular diseases and cancer, Alzheimer's is the third-largest market in the world in terms of cost of treatment of the disease, as well as the third leading cause of mortality in the industrialized world. It is hard not to imagine a fit population of baby boomers turning the

Alzheimer's curve around, recapturing those billions, and redirecting them for other beneficial purposes.

PARKINSON'S DISEASE

Nearly a million people in the United States are currently afflicted with Parkinson's disease, and more than 50,000 are diagnosed with it each year. This degenerative disorder of the central nervous system impairs motor skills and speech primarily and has no known cure. Drug therapies only treat the symptoms. In Parkinson's, cells in the brain that contain dopamine, a neurotransmitter essential for muscle control, progressively die until only a small percentage remains. Dopamine carries signals along nerve fibers that end in the part of the brain involved in control of movement. In the absence of dopamine, neurons can't send the appropriate messages for smooth motor control, resulting in the telltale symptoms of Parkinson's: uncontrollable tremors, rigidity of limbs, slow movements, and stooped posture.

It is a disease that usually affects people over the age of 50. Typically, the disease begins around the age of 60. However, there have been increasing reports of "early-onset" Parkinson's disease in recent years, and it has been estimated that 5 to 10 percent of sufferers are under the age of 40. Actor Michael J. Fox was 30 when he was diagnosed with the disease.

Scientists from the Harvard School of Public Health, University of Pittsburgh, and University of Southern California have been finding that exercise might offer a powerful defense against the onset of Parkinson's. Their studies suggest physical activity might help protect neurons in the brain from the ongoing damage of Parkinson's, leading one researcher to remark that a daily run might do what drugs have been unable to, so far.

At the University of Pittsburgh, researchers found that exercise offered rats a powerful shield against a Parkinson's-like disease. At the same time they were put on a strenuous exercise regimen, the rats were injected with a toxin that kills brain cells, yet they never developed symptoms and had almost no sign of damage to the brain, including to the dopamine-producing neurons. The study concluded that exercise almost completely protected against the loss of those neurons.

The Harvard study in 2005, conducted at the Harvard School of Public Health, concluded that men who had been runners, played basketball, or did some other strenuous physical activity at least twice a week as young adults reduced their risk of getting Parkinson's later by 60 percent. People who are healthy now are advised to build a serious fitness routine into their daily schedule. Play basketball. Run. Bicycle. Swim laps.

The advice is much the same for people who have the disease. Experts say running, walking, and other activities all help build muscle mass, which is a boon for people who are fighting not just the disease but also the loss of muscle power that comes with increasing age. People who exercise regularly may be less likely to develop Parkinson's disease—but leisurely strolls won't be sufficient. All the indicators point to the need for a higher level of energy output than merely walking.

Harvard researchers reported that the most important thing learned from this study was that high levels of moderate to vigorous recreational physical activity (like biking, swimming, aerobics, etc.) were associated with lower Parkinson's disease risk. Participants with the highest levels of physical activity at the beginning of the study had a notably lower risk of getting the disease over the next ten years than those with low levels of activity or none at all.

People who reported the highest levels of recreational physical activity in the study were reportedly doing about the equivalent of 5–6 hours of aerobics or 3–4 hours of lap swimming each week. Their Parkinson's disease risk was 40 percent lower than the people who reported no physical activity, or only light activities like walking. Level of intensity and the amount of time spent each week were the deciding criteria.

Exercise has the added benefit of giving people with Parkinson's greater strength, which leads to better balance. Fitter patients are more functional, and better able to perform daily tasks that can help keep them independent.

STRESS

Stress is one of those conditions that has been labeled a "silent killer" of our time, a consequence of the frenetic pace of contemporary life, where few of us are ever free from sources of pressure and anxiety. The demands of daily life in today's world are unprecedented, and we are all challenged to find ways of managing stress. The statistics are staggering. Two-thirds of Americans admit that they are likely to seek help for combating stress. Our epidemic of depression and anxiety disorders has enabled a multibillion-dollar industry of pharmaceuticals to help people cope with the stresses that seem so much a part of modern lifestyles.

Successful centenarians tend to be successful not only at avoiding major diseases and debilitation, but also at coping with stress. As we saw in Chapter 6, optimism, hope, and the ability to cope with loss are hallmarks of the psychological profile of a long healthy life. These are all components of a healthy stress management program. Mme. Calment, our 122-year-old archetype, seems to have been exemplary in this regard, since she was fully engaged with life and surely had to navigate her way through any number of stress-inducing situations long after passing the century mark.

The term "stress" in its current psychological meaning was coined by famed endocrinologist Hans Selye, who then gave us the General

Adaptation Syndrome to describe its physiological consequences; the syndrome is largely reducible to the "fight or flight" response.

Exposure to stress and the stress hormone corticosterone has been shown to decrease the production of BDNF in rats, and if the stress levels persist, can lead to an eventual atrophy of the hippocampus. Atrophy of the hippocampus and other deep-brain structures has been shown to take place in humans suffering from extended periods of chronic depression.

It is widely believed that memory impairment associated with aging is caused by damage to the hippocampus as a result of lifelong exposure to stress hormones. Several studies have shown that elderly people with significant and prolonged elevation of these stress hormones have smaller hippocampal regions and show declines in memory due to damage to the hippocampus. Reducing stress hormone levels in aged rats can restore the production rate of brain cells in the hippocampus.

All forms of stress produce the same physiological consequences. This includes environmental stress (for example, heat, cold, noise), chemical stress (pollution, drugs, etc.), physical stress (overexertion, exhaustion, trauma, infection), psychological stress (anxiety, fear, shock), and biochemical stress (nutritional deficiencies, dietary excesses, refined sugar consumption, etc.). All of these different sources of stress are cumulative in their effects.

Stress is the gateway to a broad spectrum of health issues. Compromised immune response is perhaps the most pernicious, and various studies have linked stress to nearly every condition in the medical encyclopedia. Simply avoiding stress is not a realistic strategy in today's world, and in fact stress is integral to our nature, our biology. What is important is how we metabolize stress, how we incorporate our ability to deal with it in our daily lives in order to avoid the latter stages of Selye's General Adaptation Syndrome—exhaustion, burnout, and, in extreme cases, death.

Interviews with centenarians tend to be largely narratives of appreciation for the life they've had and been able to enjoy, not chronicles of unhappiness, trauma, conflict, or despair. There is an unequivocal connection between successful stress management and successful long-term living. Which brings us to the all-important concept of attitude. It is tempting to label attitude an intangible because we can't quantify it, but a positive attitude, an embracing of each day of life, is a psychological glue that binds both health and longevity. A healthy attitude is a survivor's attitude.

CHAPTER 9

FOOD AND NUTRITION

A life span of 100 years, assuming an average of 3 meals per day, adds up to a total of around 110,000 meals. At 2,000 calories per day, that's about 75 million calories in total, an enormous energy metric, a staggering amount of food. The energetic requirements of a human life are impressive.

Looking back at our species' history, we see that we have been either underfed or overfed virtually the entire time. Our time as hunter-gatherers, more than 99 percent of our accumulated history, was characterized by widespread starvation. Even in more recent times, famines have ravaged entire populations.

Rather suddenly, however, we have turned the tables on this phenomenon with a vengeance. Globesity, a term coined by the World Health Organization (WHO), is the new crisis, threatening to suppress the life expectancy curve of future generations. For the first time in history, our planet holds more overfed than underfed people. Obesity has, in many quarters, become the nutritional norm. It has been noted that half of what we now eat keeps us living; the other half keeps the doctors living well!

It is hard to imagine a subject more riddled with confusion, contradiction, and misinformation than that of food and nutrition. Here in the twenty-first century it seems absurd that we don't have a firmer grip on what constitutes optimum food intake for health and longevity. We are awash in information, some of it conflicting, much of it simply unsound, with regular surprises as we learn that yesterday's miracle food (or supplement) is now out of favor or bad for you! Carbohydrates are in and then they're out. No-fat diets are in and then they're out. Meat is bad for you—or is it? Beta-carotene prevents cancer—or maybe it actually causes it! Who knows for sure? What appears to be a matter of common sense often turns out to be counterintuitive.

A recent search of the Amazon book list reveals 23,000 titles concerning diet. It would be a fair guess to estimate that most of the nutritional science claimed by the authors is gimmicky and ultimately wrong. A calorie is a calorie is a calorie. A calorie is a very specific measure of energy, the amount of heat required to raise one cubic centimeter of water by one degree. A calorie of fat has the same amount of energy as a calorie of protein or carbohydrate. All weight gain and weight loss, over time, is a strict calculation based on caloric intake. Weight gain and weight loss are the ultimate measure of amount and not type. Theoretically it is possible to gain weight eating lettuce, if you eat enough; so too it is possible to lose weight eating lard, if taken in small amounts. Similarly, Dr. Bortz has shown that the timing of calories does not affect their disposition. In "The Effect of Feeding Frequency on Rate of Weight Loss," published in the *New England Journal of Medicine,* popular misconceptions about food intake at different times of day or night are shown to be largely insupportable. On average, it really doesn't matter.

It's reasonable to wonder why there isn't greater universal consensus about dietary guidelines. After all, we live in a period of luminary science, when we can measure objects practically at the outer limits of the universe and compute quantum-level properties to one part in 10^{15}. Surely we should be able to reduce nutrition to an exact science!

"Reduce" suggests reductionism, of course, which is the eye of the nutrition hurricane. If there is one area of health that is surely more than the sum of its parts, it would be nutrition. At least as far back as ancient Egypt, we have sought in our sources of food and drink that magic potion, the blessed fruit, the fountain of youth, the special formula that would keep us young and healthy. It's a pursuit that continues unabated today.

What should we be eating? The extraordinary variety of diets that constitute the daily fare of the globe's 300 million people is a testament to our amazing versatility as a species. We are truly omnivores, and the study of our nutritional biochemistry reveals the depth of our "metabolic pool." Digestion of each of our foodstuffs—whether it be carbohydrates, fats, or proteins—ultimately yields the same molecular product, acetyl CoA, which is then either combusted for energy or synthesized to fat, our storage bin for excess calories.

The "food pyramid" that we have all seen in one form or another has evolved considerably over the decades and continues to generate controversy in many quarters, indicating how thorny the subject can be. The U.S. Department of Agriculture has been publishing food guides periodically since 1916, with the most recent version coming out in 2005. Along the way, there has been radical evolution, eventually differentiating protein sources, fats, sugars, types of vegetables, and oils. Even today the model invites controversy. A group at the Harvard School of Public Health took issue with shortcomings in the science behind the USDA model and produced their own, with the intention of employing only the best contemporary science, as found in peer-reviewed scientific journals. It departs from its predecessors by having a non-food base of exercise and weight control, and includes calcium and multi-vitamin supplements as well as alcohol in moderate amounts.

Even so, the Harvard model has been criticized. In their book *Fantastic Voyage: Live Long Enough to Live Forever,* published in 2004, Ray

Kurzweil and Terry Grossman, M.D, point out that the guidelines provided in the Harvard pyramid fail to distinguish between healthy and
unhealthy oils. In addition, whole-grain foods are given more priority
than vegetables, which should not be the case as vegetables have a lower
glycemic load (a measure of how quickly blood sugar rises in response
to a specific amount of a food taken in). Other observations are that
fish should be given a higher priority due to its high omega-3 content,
and that high-fat dairy products should be excluded. As an alternative,
the authors postulate a new food pyramid, emphasizing low glycemic
load vegetables; healthy fats, such as avocados, nuts, and seeds; lean animal protein; fish; and extra virgin olive oil.

Not satisfied with any of the others, the University of Michigan's
School of Integrative Medicine created their own, a "Healing Foods"
pyramid that emphasizes plant-based choices, variety, and balance. It
includes sections for seasonings and water as well as healthy fats.

The fact that all of this very basic information continues to spark so
much debate and difference of opinion is telling.

A major confounding factor is that so much of the science that has
been applied to food has been that same reductionist approach that we
have taken issue with in earlier chapters. We know a great deal about the
nutritional needs of our bodies and can easily come up with an extensive list of the minerals, vitamins, elements, and compounds that are required to sustain the operation of a healthy body. The problem is that

when we try to separate out those nutritional elements from the total process of sustaining our metabolic processes, we find that the sum of the parts doesn't come close to adding up to the effect of the whole. An excellent example of this is the study that found the total health benefits of whole grains could not be accounted for by simply adding up the benefits attributable to each of the nutritional elements in the grain.

The process of digestion gets insufficient consideration for its role as mediator between what we put in our mouth and what ends up as life-sustaining material at our vital organs. Digestion is the chemical process that breaks down the contents of our stomach into smaller and smaller units, until there are sufficiently small molecules to allow transport through the tissues and into the bloodstream. Carbohydrates, for example, spend the least amount of time in the stomach, while protein stays in the stomach longer, and fats the longest. As the food dissolves into the various secretions of the pancreas, liver, and intestine, the contents of the intestine are mixed and pushed forward to allow further digestion. A great many chemical changes take place in this process. Together, nerves, hormones, the blood, and the organs of the digestive system conduct the complex tasks of digesting and absorbing nutrients from the foods and liquids you consume each day.

Food is, of course, more complex than merely a source of fuel. It is a major source of pleasure, of psychic comfort, an expression of tribal identification; we have as complicated a relationship with food as we do with anything in our lives. Why do people persist in consuming things that are unhealthy and bad for them? One might as well ask why people continue to have bad relationships, even though they know better.

But there is no reason for us to add to the confusion or deepen the complexity about food and nutrition issues. We can assert a few simple rules, and the reader might simply skip ahead after reading them, or stick around for the details.

Michael Pollan's landmark book, *In Defense of Food*, sets forth a simple philosophy about eating that contains essential wisdom. It states, with understated power: Eat food, mostly plants, not too much. This simple mantra contains sufficient information to guide us on the path to a century of healthy eating.

The term "eat food" is meant provocatively to distinguish natural food from the sum of its nutrient elements. As noted above with the example of whole grains, when we try to reduce food to its component parts, we find that our bodies simply don't recognize the sum of those parts for their whole. Our reductionist tradition has conditioned us to expect a formulaic approach to nutrition, as it has to other sciences. That is, we know that we require so many grams of proteins, carbohydrates, and fats; so many units of the various vitamins; so many milligrams of essential minerals. Why not simply create a nutrition pill that contains all those essential elements, and guarantee ourselves a program of bulletproof healthy nutrition? Science fiction has a long tradition, in fact, of postulating just such a scenario.

The fact is that we are the products of our evolutionary heritage, and for nearly 99 percent of the time that genus *homo* has inhabited the planet, we have subsisted largely on whole grains, leaves and roots, fruits, nuts and berries, with occasional animal protein. Radical departures challenge our natural ability to process food effectively and keep our internal engines running smoothly. It is bad enough that we acquired a taste for refined grains and sugars. The example of Wonder Bread will probably be noted by future historians as a turning point in nutritional nonsense, where so many of the essential ingredients of the grain had been removed that the manufacturer made a major promotional issue of all the vitamins and minerals that had to be added back in—none of which really altered the nutritional value of the product appreciably.

Context is critical when it comes to nutrition. Our stores and fast food chains present an array of products that pass muster as food largely on the strength of added ingredients, often synthetic vitamins and minerals that are not an inherent part of the original food product. The failure of this approach is all around us in the epidemic of obesity and diabetes that is generally considered to derive from "the western diet." It is this evolution of eating patterns that has been ruinous to a large segment of our population today.

THE CARNIVORE CONUNDRUM

Meat has been an ongoing source of controversy for decades. We seem to know almost intuitively that vegetables are somehow "healthier" for us than meats, but we have a distinct need for protein in our diets and meats are—and have been for millennia—a ready source of protein. Now, however, there is new evidence definitively showing how eating quantities of red and processed meat damages health. These negative impacts are seen particularly with "marbled" or fatty meat, which is generally considered the most flavorful and hence desirable.

Researchers from the U.S. National Cancer Institute followed more than 500,000 people over a ten-year period, and found that big meat eaters had a markedly increased risk of death from all causes. Those whose diet contained the highest proportion of red or processed meat had a higher overall risk of death, and specifically a higher risk of cancer and heart disease, than those who ate the least. People eating the most meat were eating about 160g of red or processed meat per day—equivalent to a daily 6-oz steak. Those who ate the least were only getting about 25g of meat per day, or the equivalent of a single slice of bacon. The researchers calculated that 11 percent of deaths in men and 16 percent of deaths in women during the study period could have been prevented if people had decreased their red meat consumption to the level of those in the lowest intake group.

There are several sources of health issues with meat. Researchers in this study cited the formation of carcinogens when cooking red meat at high temperatures as a primary example. Meat is also rich in saturated fats, which are linked with colorectal and breast cancers. Protein is not stored in the body, and protein intake that is not immediately used is flushed out with urine, adding stress to the kidneys. Additionally, other studies have shown that lowering meat intake results in lower risk of heart disease, as well as improved blood pressure and cholesterol levels.

The majority opinion today does not, however, advocate a meatless diet. Fresh lean red meat is a good source of protein and other nutrients, and we have evolved as omnivores, after all. The issue is one of quantity and proportion. Most Americans today would be well advised to reduce their consumption of red meat considerably. Between 30 and 60g per day has been a figure suggested by research as a safe number that is least likely to tip the scales toward cancer or heart disease (note that 60g is just slightly more than 2 ounces). Processed, highly salted meats, on the other hand, find little to recommend them in any quantity because there is so little health benefit against a high risk of negative consequences.

Fish, on the other hand, has become a more frequent source of study in recent years, and evidence continues to mount in favor of the health-enhancing value of increasing the consumption of fish as an alternative to other animal sources. In addition to its value as a source of protein,

various studies have consistently found a correlation between fish consumption and lower risk of dementia. Researchers found that among
nearly 15,000 older adults living in China, India, and several Latin
American countries, the odds of having dementia generally declined as
fish consumption rose. For each increase in participants' reported fish
intake—from never, to some days of the week, to most or all days of the
week—the incidence of dementia dropped by nearly 20 percent. The
findings also determined that the fish-dementia link does not simply
reflect the benefits of a generally higher-quality diet. The study found
that adults who ate the most meat were more likely to have dementia
than those who never ate meat.

It is generally thought that much of the benefit from eating fish
comes primarily from the omega-3 fatty acids found most abundantly in
oily fish like salmon, mackerel, and albacore tuna. Lab studies show that
omega-3 fats have a number of properties that could help stave off dementia—including actions that protect nerve cells, limit inflammation,
and help prevent the buildup of the amyloid proteins seen in the brains
of Alzheimer's patients. The relationship between higher fish intake
and lower dementia prevalence was consistent across all countries, with
the exception of India. The link also held when the researchers factored
in participants' incomes, education, and lifestyle habits like smoking and
fruit and vegetable intake—suggesting that differences in socioeco-
nomics do not fully account for the finding.

The recent popularity of omega-3 as a broad-spectrum health aid has led to an increasing number of studies focusing on its properties and its actual benefits. Not surprisingly, many of the studies are finding inconclusive evidence about the claims made by its adherents with respect to issues beyond general cardiovascular health, and optimum dosages are still not entirely well known; nonetheless, the case for eating fish vs. red meat appears to be no contest. The one concern about fish is the presence of mercury, which can accumulate in the flesh over time and with the growth of the fish. Fortunately, only a few popular fish can be characterized as having higher levels of it, including swordfish, ahi tuna, orange roughy, and shark. On the low end, and of no concern to the mercury conscious, are such regular fare as crab, clams, shrimp, anchovies, salmon, trout, sole, squid, oysters, tilapia, sardines, and herring.

The example of red meat serves to point up the wisdom in Pollan's third admonition, "not too much." Earlier, we cited the Delphic Oracle's advice to know thyself. The other advisory handed down by the Oracle some 3,000 years ago is "moderation in all things." We are notorious over-consumers, largely because of the accessibility and relatively cheap cost of calorically dense food products. Even so, one must ask: Why do we do this? Why so little resistance to the consumption of processed foods with their fats and oils, high-fructose corn sugar, salt, and chemical additives, knowing that it's bad for us in so many ways?

The answer is embedded in our genome, its origins in our primeval legacy. In nature, animals that don't die from predation by other animals generally starve to death. Starvation is nature's grim reaper, and most of the narrative of animal life centers on the struggle to avoid starvation. So it was with our primitive antecedents. Paleolithic man's life was driven by hunger, and when a caloric surplus was available, he availed himself of the opportunity. Accumulating fat stores has always been a hedge against an early demise, and until recent history, putting on surplus poundage was considered a boon to health, not a threat.

These life-preserving urges remain with us today and help explain why a hamburger loaded with fats and salt on a bun of refined carbohydrates would usually be chosen over, say, an apple by a hungry person. We still feel the tug of our ancestral motives to feast when the opportunity presents itself. But now, many millennia later, we have choices beyond feast or famine. The challenge is to recast our thinking and recognize the consequences of our choices.

The theme of moderation crops up in almost every study of population groups with an unusually high percentage of centenarians. One of the most common factors among the diets of centenarians is not only the consumption of good foods, but also the practice of eating small amounts of food over the course of the day. The longevity benefit of consuming smaller amounts of food has been well known from studies on caloric restriction.

Researchers from Mount Sinai School of Medicine have done extensive animal studies on the physiological reasons behind the concept that dietary restriction leads to lower incidence of age-related diseases and increased longevity, while over-consumption leads to the opposite. Initial results from this study showed that following a diet about 30 percent lower in calories than a typical one led to an optimal level of reduction in development of age-related conditions like Alzheimer's disease, as well as slowed the aging process, increasing life span by about 50 percent among the test animals. Interestingly, it appears that how the diet is restricted—by reducing fats, proteins, carbohydrates, etc.—is inconsequential. A 10 percent reduction in calories led to only a slight increase in life span. Conversely, the researchers found that a high-calorie diet has a tendency to accelerate age-related disease by promoting oxidative stress and increasing the odds against a longer life span.

Radical caloric restriction almost certainly extends life, but at what price? It should not be necessary to starve yourself in order to enjoy a longer life. We have ample examples, as well as studies on laboratory animals, that show how moderate consumption of good foods, spaced smartly over the course of the day, can be a bulwark of a healthy lifestyle and a key ally on the road to a very long life.

On the island of Okinawa, where there are more centenarians per capita than anywhere else in the world, diet is a prominent and distinguishing lifestyle feature. The typical Okinawan diet is dominated by whole grains, vegetables, and fish, with little or no eggs, meat, or dairy products. Okinawans are probably one of the world's largest consumers of tofu on a per-capita basis. Soy products have enjoyed a reputation for health-modulating effects because soy is particularly rich in flavonoids, which have strong antioxidant properties. But most likely a key factor is that Okinawans tend to follow a philosophy of specific moderation when it comes to food consumption. Rather than stopping when they feel full, they eat only to the point at which they feel about 80 percent full. They have a name for this practice, *hara hachi bu,* which literally translates to "eight parts out of ten."

This practice lends credence to the free-radical theory of aging, since a calorically reduced diet presents fewer opportunities for the formation of free radicals in the process of metabolism. Studies on older Okinawans reveal consistently low blood levels of free radicals. The same studies found impressively youthful clean arteries and low cholesterol. It should be noted that Okinawans also enjoy regular exercise at all ages, moderate alcohol consumption, avoidance of smoking, and a psycho-spiritual character that minimizes stress.

We can assert the importance of diet and cite numerous other populations with a high percentage of centenarians and draw conclusions from their dietary patterns. However, every example will also be characterized by other key variables, particularly exercise. For instance, Azerbaijan also has very impressive longevity statistics. In the last census

Azerbaijan claimed nearly 50 people over the age of 100 out of every 100,000 residents, or about 15,000 centenarians in total. Against conventional wisdom, and contrary to the diets of the Okinawans, the Azerbaijani diet features fatty meats and dairy products, such as milks and sour creams. While some have puzzled over this apparent anomaly, Azeri medical professionals have pointed out that the national diet has historical guidelines emphasizing balance and moderation. For instance, they have a tradition of accompanying any consumption of meat with vegetables, greens, and beans. They also consume a great deal of garlic and yogurt. Yogurt adherents like to claim extensive health and longevity benefits from its use, but to date no convincing studies have put yogurt in a life-extending category.

In an interesting footnote, Elie Metchnikoff, a Russian biologist who won the 1908 Nobel Prize, believed that the lactobacilli in yogurt were the key to major life extension. He studied the dietary habits of French, Russian, and Bulgarian peasants, and noted that the Bulgarians, who lived longer than the others, on average, consumed several liters of yogurt each day. Bypassing all the other possible differences, Metchnikoff was so impressed with the yogurt consumption that he built an entire theory on it. He embraced a personal yogurt regimen and assured everyone that he would live to 150. He died at 71, an impressively long life for a Russian male of his generation, regardless.

Similar stories to the Azerbaijanis' abound. The remote Greek island of Ikaria reportedly has the largest percentage of over-90 people
in the world, and they attribute their longevity to an herbal tea they
drink that consists of mint, rosemary, purple sage, and spleenwort.
One has to dig a bit deeper to discover that because of the rugged ter-
rain and lack of local motorized transport, locals are noted for the
amount of exercise they maintain, even well into their later years. And
their daily diet is dominated by olive oil, fruit, vegetables, and very little processed food.

The Italian island of Sardinia is also noted for its high proportion
of centenarians. Locals point to the grapes that island wines are made
from, which are especially rich in polyphenols and antioxidants. Sar-
dinians are also sustained by the classic "Mediterranean diet" rich in
olive oil, fruits and vegetables, and fish. They are also known for being
active and fit.

In the Hunza Valley in the most remote mountains of Pakistan,
people routinely live into their nineties, which researchers believe could
be due to their diet of fruit, grain, and vegetables. It should be noted
that the Hunzas have also been the source of a great deal of misinformation and opportunism, with pitches for their "longevity bread" and
"living water" from glacial runoff appearing in western health food
sources (usually bearing no honest connection to Hunza itself).

The Vilcabamba region of southern Ecuador is another area where large numbers of residents appear to reach their 100th birthday in good health. Some have tried to attribute this longevity to the consumption of a natural mineral water, which is notably free from impurities. However, scientists who have been observing the people of this region systematically since the 1950s attribute the longevity to a diet of mostly raw fruits, nuts, and vegetables, with virtually no animal products or processed food. And, yes, lifelong activity at a fairly demanding level, with daily hikes up steep slopes and the cultivation and harvest of food crops.

What can we infer from these, and other examples of isolated groups with exceptional longevity? Diet is important, to be sure. There is a dietary/nutritional story intrinsic to every one of these. But it is never the whole story. In every one of these examples, there is a matrix of factors, typically led by exercise, and after that the avoidance of unhealthy life choices, like smoking. And in most cases there are social factors, particularly strong family and community cultures.

There is no evidence whatsoever supporting the notion that one can simply eat one's way to health, much less an exceptional life span. It seems to be an essential part of human nature that we associate our wellbeing with our food intake and its corollaries, the intake of pills, medicines, and supplements, and hence look to this function so readily for solutions. In the case of legitimate nutritional deficiencies, of course, this makes perfect sense. Historically, it was probably when people began to make long sea voyages that the effects of deprivation from fresh foods were revealed in a systematic way.

Today, however, we have few excuses not to eat a complete, balanced, and fully nutritional diet. Except for pockets of poverty and isolation, most of us have the basic knowledge of and accessibility to all the foods that we need to maintain nutritional health. If we assume this to be the case, it then begs the question: Why are we a society so bombarded with exhortations to buy vitamins and a bewildering lineup of nutritional supplements?

VITAMINS, SUPPLEMENTS, AND THE WORLD'S MOST EXPENSIVE URINE

Americans spend on the order of $25 billion annually on vitamins and nutritional supplements. This is a staggering figure, particularly against the backdrop of our huge national health crisis. A case can be made that both phenomena spring from an insufficiency of nutritional knowledge.

Vitamins are another essential part of food that is absorbed through the small intestine, organic compounds that can't be synthesized within our bodies and must come from our diet. The word "vitamin" is a contraction of *vital mineral*, the term first coined with the discovery of vitamins in the early nineteenth century. The two types of vitamins are classified by the fluid in which they can be dissolved: water-soluble vitamins (all the B vitamins and vitamin C) and fat-soluble vitamins (vitamins A, D, E, and K). Fat-soluble vitamins are stored in the liver and fatty tissue of the body, whereas water-soluble vitamins are not easily stored and excess amounts are flushed out in the urine.

The only reason to take a vitamin is if you have reason to believe that you are deficient in that vitamin. With only a handful of exceptions, all necessary vitamins are contained in the foods we all should be eating as a routine part of our daily living, particularly those foods that form the base of all the various food pyramids: that is, fresh fruits, fresh vegetables, particularly darker green ones, nuts, and whole grains. Besides getting demonstrably better benefit from vitamins that are an integral part of your food, there is no danger of vitamin toxicity from overdosing this way. And it should go without saying that it is categorically not possible to compensate for an unhealthy diet by simply adding vitamins. Nutrition should come from the farm, not the pharmacy.

There can be exceptions. Dental problems, or social isolation, for instance, may conspire to cause a vitamin deficiency. Many surveys of large numbers of older persons regularly alert us to this "hidden" malnutrition. If a person has a specific deficiency owing to some other condition, then it makes sense to supplement with specific vitamins. Vitamin D is perhaps the best example. There are widespread defi-

ciencies in D, especially among older people who get outside infrequently and who may have inadequate diets, and a research study across
65,000 test subjects showed that strong doses of vitamin D (400 international units or better) daily led to a reduction in the incidence of
bone fractures. Vitamin B12 is another example: It is a vitamin that
older people sometimes have trouble absorbing. Is there any benefit for
a person over 60, say, in taking a simple multi-vitamin pill on a daily
basis? It's possible. And it does no harm, so why not?

It is not uncommon to find health-conscious people with drawers
full of vitamins and supplements that they take every day, as well as having a good, balanced, thoroughly nutritious diet. It is for these people
that the phrase "the world's most expensive urine" was coined. Put simply, massive doses of vitamins add nothing to one's health or longevity.
There is not a single legitimate study showing otherwise.

It is bad enough that vitamins are misconstrued and misused as a
nutritional element. What is far worse are the abuses of vitamins as potential preventive or curative agents of major diseases that are not the
result of a dietary deficiency, particularly cardiovascular diseases and
cancers. We have an abundance of recent studies that have looked for a
link between vitamin supplementation and major diseases, and the results have been uniformly negative. An eight-year study of multi-
vitamin use among 16,000 older women as part of the Women's Health

Initiative found no reduction in the risk of cancer or heart disease in this group as a result of the extra vitamin intake. Another study around the same time tracked 15,000 men for ten years. One group took extra vitamin C and E, and the others took a placebo. Both groups came up with identical results. Also in the same time period, 35,000 men were studied for the effects of high doses of vitamin E and selenium on lowering the risk of prostate cancer. Like the other studies, this showed no correlation.

Even more damning, a 2007 paper in the *Journal of the American Medical Association* reviewed mortality rates in randomized trials of antioxidant supplements and found a 5 percent increase in mortality among the groups taking the supplements! Nobel laureate and "father of molecular biology" Linus Pauling's megadose theory of vitamin C that launched much of the current vogue for supplemental vitamins may have its counterpoint in the findings that, in the laboratory, cancer cells thrive on vitamin C. Vitamin C is also found in higher levels in tumors than in normal tissue.

Vitamin E, which has been a darling of the health profession as well as the health conscious in general for decades now, has been particularly savaged by the latest research. A German study team found that vitamin E had a negative effect in conjunction with exercise because it tended to suppress the body's natural oxidative defense mechanisms after a workout. Other tests have found virtually no discernible benefit to taking vitamin E in supplemental pill form and, in fact, found that typical popular dosages of 400 international units actually *increased* mortality rates.

We are awash in promotions for antioxidants, and a stroll through any health food store might give one the impression that the great medical challenge of our times is the battle against free radicals and their oxidative effects. It's possible to draw the conclusion that if one simply ate enough pomegranate, blueberry, and açai berry (pick your favorite antioxidant source du jour), one ought to be all but immortal. But it doesn't work that way.

First, we really don't have to look that far or that hard to find convenient sources of antioxidants. Literally every fresh vegetable and fruit is laden with antioxidant compounds, not just a handful of specialized species. A single leaf of thyme contains at least 35 known antioxidants. It is safe to say that if you eat fresh fruit and vegetables every day, you will get all the antioxidants your body can put to effective use. It is that simple.

According to the Antioxidants Laboratory at the Human Nutrition Research Center on Aging at Tufts University, there are on the order of 20,000 different antioxidants in a good diet. Director Jeffrey Blumberg has been quoted as noting that "There aren't 20,000 pills to take. One of the reasons dietary supplements can't replace a healthful diet is because we don't know about what's important to put in every pill."

THE MYTHOLOGY OF
NUTRITIONAL SUPPLEMENTS

Virtually every shopping mall of any size in America has a health food store peddling supplements and vitamins. Most modern supermarkets have racks of the same. And yet one doesn't have to dig very deep to see that there is a near consensus among professionals that almost all of these are worthless.

Under the Dietary Supplement and Health Education Act of 1994, nutritional supplements do not have to be tested for safety or effectiveness before going on the market. As long as the manufacturer doesn't claim that a product treats or cures a specific disease, it can tout any health benefit it has the nerve to. The current glut of products that promise to "strengthen your immune system" are a blatant example. Considerable laboratory testing has been done on widely available supplements, and the findings are invariably shocking. A great many don't contain what they claim to, or in the amounts they claim to have. Many contain filler material that is potentially dangerous. It is important for people to understand how little regulatory scrutiny these products have. For instance, one recent study of 59 different commercial echinacea supplements found that nearly half contained no echinacea at all. This is not unusual.

But perhaps even more important is the fact that nearly all of them do absolutely no good at all. There are perhaps a handful that have shown some utility in clinical trials, but even then the results have been modest and usually come with cautionary notes. Ginkgo biloba, for instance, has yielded some improvement in cognitive performance, but not without some conflicting data. The Ginkgo Evaluation of Memory study, the largest of its kind, indicated that it had no effect in decreasing the incidence of dementia or Alzheimer's disease in the elderly.

Glucosamine, in the form of glucosamine sulfate, has shown modest effectiveness in treating joint pain, particularly osteoarthritis of the knee. However, the older the patient and the longer the duration of the arthritis, the less effective it seems to be. It is often paired with chondroitin, which has yet to yield effective results in clinical studies.

Coenzyme Q10 is a very popular supplement at the moment, though its effects have been modest. The National Cancer Institute has expressed its concern that its safety and its effectiveness have yet to be satisfactorily determined.

Resveratrol is of particular interest because of its current high visibility and proliferation of product offerings. More than any other drug or supplement on the market today, it is being heavily touted as an "anti-aging" solution. Found in the skins of wine grapes (and also, by the way, in peanuts, spruce, eucalyptus, and mulberries, among others), resveratrol has a variety of antioxidant properties and appears to mimic the effects of caloric restriction in laboratory animals. There have been no clinical trials in human beings, and the animal results suggest that un-realistically large doses would be required in humans to have a marked effect on longevity.

This is not to say that important advances won't be found through sources like these. After all, most of the drugs in the repertoire of con-temporary doctors came from natural sources, not unlike resveratrol, glucosamine, and ginkgo. At this time there are extensive research proj-ects in tropical forests seeking out the next generation of biochemical products that will enhance our health and well-being. But those that will prove useful will do so by way of rigorous clinical testing that will de-termine not only the efficacy of the compound but also the safe dosage and the cautionary side effects, and will establish them within a regula-tory framework designed to protect the unwary consumer.

So much of this research, it must be noted with a glimmer of irony, amounts to the medical establishment (as well as "alternative medicine" advocates) working to find ways of keeping alive those people that the western diet is making ill. How much easier it would all be if people simply ate intelligently in the first place!

CHAPTER 10

100 HEALTHY YEARS IN
14 HEALTHY CHOICES

As we chart our course through life, it is important to know what is possible. What are we capable of, and what can we aspire to? What, in fact, is our potential?

A great body of evidence has accumulated in support of the idea that 100 healthy years (or more) *is* the human potential. By that we mean years of self-efficacy, of full-powered living, free of major disease or disorder, physically and cognitively. It should be so easy! The devil, as they say, is in the details.

If we have learned anything from the science of the past decade or so, it has been the overarching theme that health—and longevity—is mostly a matter of choice, not fate. Every day each of us makes thousands of decisions, many of them unconsciously. We are not likely to give up much of a typical day thinking about lofty concepts like how we might realize our full potential as a living, sentient organism. That concept, however, is implicit in our daily choices, regardless. The trick is to bring those choices to the fore, to make them an integral part of our daily lives until they are like breathing.

The achievement of those 100 (or more) healthy years is the end product of a handful of lifestyle choices based on incontrovertible science, which we have reviewed in detail in the previous chapters. If one could write a prescription that best recapitulates these accumulated findings, it would read something like this:

1. Be a realist. Aging is inevitable. It is not a disease to be cured. The second law of thermodynamics is The Law, and we are beholden to it. But accepting the inevitability of aging doesn't mean that one has to give in to it passively. All aging isn't equal. It's not as bad as you may have thought, and in fact can be nearly invisible, especially if you apply the next set of "rules." Reality is largely within each of our span of control to reshape in a great many ways.

2. Pay attention to your body. "Know thyself." The Delphic Oracle wisely gave us the first rule of a long, healthy life. Get to know your body, your internal workings, better. Pay attention to what your body is telling you. Marvel at its intricacies. Learn as much

as you can about it—don't rely on your doctor to tell you the things you should know about yourself.

Spend a little time in front of a mirror regularly. Be critical but constructive. Evaluate yourself. A little vanity can be a good thing. Ask yourself what you can do to make yourself healthier, stronger, more fit. Challenge Mother Nature.

3. Move! Move whatever is movable. Rejoice in your gift of movement. Walk. Run. Fidget. Put your joints to work. Jump (when was the last time you jumped?). Bend. Stretch. Throw your arms over your head. Swim. Play ball. Any kind of ball.

    Movement is life. The absence of movement is the absence of life. Movement should never be thought of as a chore, but as an opportunity. Our ability to move is a measure of our mastery of the space we inhabit. It is a marvelous gift. Revel in it.

4. Get strong. And stay strong. Work out with weights or an equivalent form of resistance training. Tune in to all your muscles. Embrace them, be proud of them, these amazing life helpers. Challenge them. Be strong enough to live to I00. Strength = life. Be as strong as you can be. You cannot be too strong.

5. Become a systems thinker. Learn to think in terms of your whole and not just your parts. Avoid the fallacy of thinking that one course of action will make up for the others you bypass. Be conscious of the cooperation and integration between your parts—

your organs, your muscles and bones, your sense of well-being. Beware the "magic bullet" fallacy.

6. Get fit and stay fit. Aerobic fitness must become a mantra, a way of life. It's easier than you think and virtually addictive when you get into it. Do something genuinely aerobic at least three times a week. Five would be better. Run, if you can. Appreciate the fact that you can! If you can't run, walk. Walk at every opportunity. Every day. There is no such thing as too much walking. Aerobic fitness is the best single defense against most of the cruel ravages of "default aging," from major diseases to frailty.

7. Pull yourself together. Employ self-fulfilling body language. Stand up straight. Shoulders back. Chest out. Chin up. Carry yourself young. Defy gravity. Believe in the self-fulfilling prophecy—a youthful posture will support youthful self-imagery and attitude. It is subtle but effective.

8. Eat smart. Get your nutrients from your food. Think about what you are putting in your body. There is no excuse not to. You cannot go wrong with fruits and vegetables. If your primary food source comes from plants, you have established an important beachhead on the path to a long, healthy life.

9. All things in moderation. This is 3,000-year-old wisdom from the Delphic Oracle. It's the very essence of common sense. Food? Drink? Things that are "bad for you"? A little bit won't hurt you.

We're not that fragile. These things shouldn't be sources of anxiety. Our species didn't get to the top of the evolutionary heap by being excessively fragile.

10. Don't wait for a miracle. Don't gamble on the "youth pill" even if you're feeling lucky. The odds are stacked severely against the likelihood that life-extending drugs are anywhere on the horizon. It's not going to happen. Medical science isn't going to make the antidote for your lifestyle poisons. The sooner you liberate yourself from this notion, the better your odds.

11. Forget about your genes. Good genes, bad genes? Forget about it. No matter what's in your personal genome, it will never be the dominant factor in your personal outcome. The very point of being human is that ability to carve out our personal destiny. Again, the state of your life and your health is a matter of choice, not fate.

12. Be necessary. Be engaged. But it's even better to be *necessary*, to have a defining sense of purpose. The life-affirming and life-extending power of this intangible factor is incalculable. Invest your relationships with value and meaning. Think of your family and friends as your personal convoy escorting you through the passage of your life.

13. Celebrate your sexuality. The great majority of discussions of aging health completely overlook sex. Perhaps it's because sex

generally is still a subject that many are uncomfortable discussing or even acknowledging. But our sexuality has great life-giving and life-restoring power, and is such an integral part of our life's engine, our motive force. We are capable of enjoying sex indefinitely, and when we do, we add healthy, vital years to our lives.

14. Go for the flow. We all intuitively know what the "flow" is. It's when everything meshes, when all the components of a system come together in perfect harmony, and we seem to be in a place where everything seems to require no effort. Athletes sometimes refer to "being in the zone," when everything is working and they seem to be at the top of their form. That is flow. Musicians and artists experience flow when they feel as if they have merged with their work in a state of complete absorption.

A flow state ensues when one is engaged in self-controlled, goal-related, meaningful actions. With health, flow can be a constant state and not just a chain of certain moments. Flow is the expression of optimum health, a convergence of aerobic fitness, strength, engagement, nutrition, attitude, outlook, and sexual energy. In the sense that we are using it here, the concept of flow has been articulated by the University of Chicago psychologist Mihaly Csikszentmihalyi as a field of behavioral science examining connections between satisfaction and daily activities. It is the embodiment of "peak experience" that is both rewarding and demanding; demanding because, once experienced, it creates a standard that one will always feel compelled to uphold.

Aristotle observed 2,300 years ago that, more than anything, men and women seek happiness, and thought that it was best expressed in terms of the Golden Mean, an idealized state between two extremes. Flow can be thought of in this context, a phenomenon that occurs at the idealized intersection of capacity and task, of organism and environment. That is, flow occurs when challenge and capacity intersect. When challenge exceeds perceived capacity, stress is the result. When opportunity is less than capacity, boredom ensues.

Flow never occurs in a static environment; it is associated with purposeful activity. In this sense we can then say that flow contains all the parameters that make up physical health. *Mens sana in corpore sano,* all is harmony.

THE ROLE OF MEDICINE

The theme of this book has been not just a blueprint for achieving a long life, but the underlying subtext of reclaiming ownership of one's health. A great part of the blame for the woeful condition of our national health care lies with the tendency to look to the medical establishment—our institutions, clinics, physicians, and the pharmaceutical industry—for all of our answers. In fact, we have a tendency to assume, in a de facto way, that the medical establishment owns our health, that it is our doctors' responsibility to find ways to keep us healthy and alive, regardless of our behaviors. This is, of course, all wrong. Medicine is still woefully disease-centric rather than health-centric.

We envision a new order in medicine in which the medical profession creates a new cadre of practitioners out of our medical schools who are health specialists rather than disease specialists. In the meantime, however, medicine has a specific range of functions that will help ever more of us attain that pinnacle of 100 healthy years.

Medicine must continue to intervene in the prevention and cure of infectious and congenital diseases; this is modern medicine's greatest triumph to date, and it must continue to progress. Many infectious diseases are like booby traps on our path to 100, and medicine should continue to do battle with these.

Medical research must continue to play a vital role in understanding pathogens and their dynamics and finding ways of dealing with them. It must also provide deeper science into our genetic makeup and further our understanding of the biochemistry of our physical processes. But we must not depend on the medical establishment for our health; ultimately, we must take ownership of and long-term responsibility for our own individual health. That is the critical step on the path to 100 healthy years.

Medicine must also rise to the challenge presented by the so-called alternative medical channels that now represent a multibillion-dollar market. More than a third of all Americans use some form of alternative health remedies. This despite the fact that virtually all of them, from acupuncture to aromatherapy, to a plethora of herbal treatments, have yet to demonstrate effectiveness in a scientific, controlled test environment—that is, double-blind, placebo-controlled studies conducted under the auspices of accredited scientists.

We are a nation increasingly—and encouragingly—concerned with health, fitness, and healthy aging. Certainly our expenditures for all forms of medical care, from conventional to alternative, from pharmaceuticals to nutritional supplements, speak well of our awareness and intentions. The solutions to the big questions, however, are strikingly inexpensive and accessible. Most of the cost is simply the intangible expense of personal energy and the willingness to embrace the life that we have evolved to enjoy.

ON LOSS AND DYING

BY WALTER BORTZ

One of my most meaningful mottos was given by my father in his adaptation of one of Robert Browning's poems, "Rabbi Ben Ezra."

Dad's words:

Then welcome each rebuff

That turns earth's smoothness rough.

That bids each man not sit, nor stand

But go

I cannot begin to recount the numerous times when these words bucked me up.

They were among the last words that I said to Dad when he was dying. They have seen me through crises that I found unbearable, only to emerge on the other side intact and probably better for the encounter.

The observation that suicide is a permanent answer to a usually temporary problem puts the time dimension in excellent perspective. But few of us are wise enough to understand that tomorrow offers a new start. I have always been fascinated by the fact that the Chinese language symbol for crisis and opportunity is the same.

The process of aging inevitably provides repeated evidences of decline. If this is the only message that is heard, then depression lurks nearby. But another of my personal philosophers, writer and editor Norman Cousins, wisely observed that nobody is smart enough to be a pessimist. The sun always comes up in the morning, regardless of what the naysayer may proclaim.

The process of aging vitally provides perspectives that our Paleolithic ancestors depended on for their very survival. The ancient Greeks and the ancient Chinese venerated aging because the elders had wisdom that could steer the youngsters through indiscretions.

My friends Paul Baltes, the psychologist who coined the term "successful aging," and human development pioneer Joan Erikson both concluded that wisdom is very rare and that most of the wise people of the world were old. The reason may be a consequence of neuroanatomy. The brain structure of the immature is full of nerve cells with few dendrites. It is only with the passage of time, and the lessons provided by experience both good and bad, that the dendrites grow, arborize, and interconnect like a shrub in springtime.

A highly personal expression of this has to do with my marathon running, which unexpectedly seems to be becoming easier the older I get. I know that I'm not going to die at mile 20, that this twitch is sure to let off in another moment or so, that the discomforts of the moment will give way to the euphoria of success before long.

A general law evolves: We become afraid of what we don't know, and with advancing years, we have fewer surprises to astound or confound us as they did when we were younger.

Irving Yalom, distinguished Stanford psychiatrist and an authority on death anxiety, in his book *Staring at the Sun,* offers a transcendent and alluring image of "ripples" as representing the eventual permanent record of each unique life. The image of ripples acknowledges the temporal nature and limitations of the physical body, but asserts the continuation of life's energies. Death in this interpretation is more than merely the shedding of our corporeal ballast; it is the persistence of our energy field. It can be thought of as a consequence of the interchangeability of matter and energy, one of the most fundamental principles of physics. The ripples concept effectively answers the primal fear of oblivion, the thought that when I die, everything about me is gone. Not so. Our ripples, the energy signature of our life, remain and endure.

Such imagery conforms to the butterfly effect of chaos theory, the idea that "thou canst not touch a flower without troubling of a star," in the poetic notion of Francis Thompson. Rippling exalts Mozart, Buddha, Aristotle, Christ, Einstein, Darwin, to name a few, whose lives' energies persist and penetrate today in a larger way than they did while alive. Similarly, even the most modest among us leaves ripples behind.

Accepting such a rich image, a philosophical, thermo-physical rendering of what death represents, can be a major breakthrough because the fear of death is at the heart of much of our anxiety. Such recognition is often catalyzed by an "awakening experience"—a dream, or loss (the death of a loved one, divorce, loss of a job or home), illness, trauma, not to mention aging. In Dr. Yalom's conception, we are encouraged to strive for more direct engagement with others. Compassionate connection enables us to overcome the terror of death and lead happier, more meaningful lives.

Once we confront our own mortality, we find it vastly easier to rearrange our priorities, communicate more deeply with those we love, appreciate more keenly the beauty of life, and increase our willingness to take the risks necessary for personal fulfillment. And imprint our ripples on the cosmos forever.

REFERENCES

CHAPTER 1

Allard, Michel, et al. *Jeanne Calment: From Van Gogh's Time to Ours, 122 Extraordinary Years.* Thorndike Senior Lifestyle (UK). A biography of the oldest documented modern centenarian, who died in 1997 at age 122.

Bortz, Walter M., M.D. "Biological Basis of Determinants of Health." *American Journal of Public Health* 95, no. 3 (March 2005). A complete definition of health is broken down into four categories, seeking to determine how much of our health is within our personal control. In this article, Dr. Bortz provides a new conceptual framework for the biological determinants of health.

Dani Sergio U., Hori A., Walter, G F (Editor), *Principles of Neural Aging* (Elsevier Science Pub., 1997). This book introduces the concept of entropy at the cellular level, not just in terms of energy flow, but in terms of its implications for information loss in cell replication as a factor in aging.

Growing Old in America: Expectations vs. Reality. Pew Research Center, June 2009. http://pewresearch.org/pubs/1269/aging-survey-expectations-versus-reality.

Hamalainen, Mark. "Thermodynamics and Information in Aging: Why Aging Is Not a Mystery and How We Will Be Able to Make Rational Interventions." *Rejuvenation Research* 8, no. 1 (Spring 2005): 29–36. doi: 10.1089/rej.2005.8.29.

Hayflick, Leonard. *How and Why We Age* (New York: Ballantine Books, 1996).

Ho, Mae-Wan. *The Rainbow and the Worm: The Physics of Organisms* (Singapore:World Scientific Publishing, 2008).

Hotz, Robert Lee. "Secrets of the Wellderly." *Wall Street Journal,* September 19, 2008. http://online.wsj.com/article/SB122176857706253591.

Hunza: A summary of the peoples of the Himalayan kingdom of Hunza whose longevity has been noted for some time now. http://longevity.about.com/od/longevitylegends/p/hunza.htm.

Okinawa Centenarians. http://www.okicent.org. Ongoing investigation of longevity among Okinawans, probably the most studied group of long-lived people anywhere.

Preamble to the Constitution of the World Health Organization as adopted by the International Health Conference, New York, June 19–22, 1946; signed on July 22, 1946, by the representatives of 61 states (Official Records of the World Health Organization, no. 2, p. 100) and entered into force on April 7, 1948.

Schneider Eric. D, and Dorion Sagan. *Into the Cool: Energy Flow, Thermodynamics and Life* (Chicago: University of Chicago Press, 2006).

Statistics on centenarians abound and have been widely offered in the media of late. See, for instance:

Bureau of the Census, *Older Americans Month: May 2009,* Facts for Features March 3, 2009, 5 pp.

The British web site http://www.thecentenarian.co.uk/AgeStatisticsCategory.html features a great deal of centenarian data and articles of interest.

Population Division, Department of Economic and Social Affairs, United Nations Secretariat, is a source of relevant global age demographics.

The Danish research study citing the probability of half the babies presently being born in the industrialized nations of the world living to 100 is the work of Professor Kaare Christensen, of the Danish Ageing Research Centre, University of Southern Denmark, Denmark, and colleagues. Results have been widely reported by news media, such as http://www.medicalnewstoday.com/articles/165960.php.

CHAPTER 2

Blair, Steven, et al. "Physical Activity, Physical Fitness, and All-Cause and Cancer Mortality: A Prospective Study of Men and Women." *Annals of Epidemiology* 6, no. 5: 452–457.

Blair, V. M., H. W. Kohl, R. S. Paffenbarger Jr., D. G. Clark, K. H. Cooper, and L. W. Gibbons. "Physical Fitness and All-Cause Mortality: A Prospective Study of Healthy Men and Women." *Journal of the American Medical Association* 262 (1989): 2395–2401.

Bortz, Walter M., M.D. "Disuse and Aging." *Journal of the American Medical Association* 248 (1982): 1203–1208. This was recently updated in: "Disuse and Aging." *The Journals of Gerontology Series A: Biological Sciences and Medical Sciences,* November 3, 2009.

Bratteby, L.-E., B. Sandhagen, and G. Samuelson. "Physical Activity, Energy Expenditure and Their Correlates in Two Cohorts of Swedish Subjects Between Adolescence and Early Adulthood." *European Journal of Clinical Nutrition* 59 (2005): 1324–1334. doi: 10.1038/sj.ejcn.1602246.

Conboy, Irina, et al. "Molecular Aging and Rejuvenation of Human Muscle Stem Cells." *EMBO Molecular Medicine,* September 30, 2009.

Fried, L. P., et al. "Frailty in Older Adults." *The Journals of Gerontology Series A: Biological Sciences and Medical Sciences* 56 (2001): M146–M157.

Guralnik, Jack M., et al. "Associations Between Lower Extremity Ischemia, Upper and Lower Extremity Strength, and Functional Impairment with Peripheral Arterial Disease." *J. Am. Geriatr. Soc.* 56, no. 4 (April 2008): 724–729.

Lee, I-Min, Chung-cheng Hsieh, and Ralph S. Paffenbarger Jr. "Exercise Intensity and Longevity in Men: The Harvard Alumni Health Study." *JAMA* 273, no. 15 (1995): 1179–1184.

Liu Y, et al. "Expression of p16INK4a in Peripheral Blood T-cells is a Biomarker of Human Aging." *Aging Cell* (4) (August 8, 2009):439–48.

Konstantinos, Nasis, et al. "Aerobic Exercise and Intraocular Pressure in Normotensive and Glaucoma Patients." *BMC Ophthalmology* 9, no. 6 (2009). doi: 10.1186/1471-2415-9-6.

Nieman D. C, Henson D A, Austin M D, Brown V A. "The immune response to a 30-minute walk." *Med Sci Sports Exerc* 37:57–62, 2005

Nurses' Health Study. http://www.channing.harvard.edu/nhs/ Paddock, Catherine. "Being Overweight Linked To "Severe Brain Degeneration"" Asreported in *MedicalNewsToday.com,* August 27, 2009. http://www.medicalnewstoday.com/articles/162135.php

Quinn, Elizabeth. "Moderate Exercise Boosts Immunity." *About.com Guide,* October 29, 2007.

Raji, Cyrus A., et al. "Brain Structure and Obesity." *Human Brain Mapping.* Spector, T. D., et al. "A Genome-Wide Association Study Identifies a Novel Locus on Chromosome 18q12.2 Influencing White Cell Telomere Length." *J. Med. Genet.* 46 (2009): 451–454. doi: 10.1136/jmg.2008.064956.

Tai-Hing Lam, et al. "Leisure Time Physical Activity and Mortality in Hong Kong: Case- Control Study of All Adult Deaths in 1998." *Annals of Epidemiology* 14, no. 6 (July 2004): 391–398.

Walston, J. et al. "Research agenda for frailty in older adults: toward a better understanding of physiology and etiology: summary from the American Geriatrics Society/National Institute on Aging Research Conference on Frailty in Older Adults." *J Am Geriatric Soc.* 2006 Jun;54(6):991–1001.

Whipple, Dan. "Paleolithic Work Ethic." *Insight on the News,* December 23, 1996. The listing of risk factors from inactivity is taken from *CureResearch.com,* http://www.cureresearch.com/risk/inactivity.htm.

Quotation from geneticist Mae-Wan Ho is from a private correspondence with Dr. Bortz. Note: The King's College (London) Department of Twin Research and Genetic Epidemiology maintains the world's largest database and study program on phenotypes from twins, effectively measuring the genetic contribution vs. environmental contribution of a great many diseases and syndromes. http://www .twin-research.ac.uk/index.html.

CHAPTER 3

Keim, Brandon. "These Toes Were Made for Running." *Wired,* February 2009. http://www.wired.com/wiredscience/2009/02/runningtoes/comment-page-2/.

Kurzweil, Ray, and Terry Grossman. *Fantastic Voyage: Live Long Enough to Live Forever* (New York: Rodale Books, 2004).

Kurzweil, Ray, and Terry Grossman. *Transcend: Nine Steps to Living Well Forever* (New York: Rodale Books, 2009).

Lloyd, D., M. A. Aon, and S. Cortassa. "Why Homeodynamics, Not Homeostasis?" *The Scientific World Journal* 1 (2001): 133–145. Mazzeo, Robert S., et al. "Exercise and Physical Activity for Older Adults." *Medicine & Science in Sports & Exercise.* 30, (6) (June 1998). http://www.acsm.org/AM/Template.cfm?Section=Past_Round-tables&Template=/CM/ContentDisplay.cfm&ContentID=2836. This paper summarizes a large number of studies correlating exercise with healthy aging.

Nieman, D. C., D. A. Henson, M. D. Austin, and V. A. Brown. "The Immune Response to a 30-Minute Walk." *Med. Sci. Sports Exerc.* 37 (2005): 57–62.

Okura, et al. "Effects of Aerobic Exercise on Metabolic Syndrome Improvement in Response to Weight Reduction." *Obesity* 15 (2007), 2478–2484; doi: 10.10308/oby.2007.294

Strohman, Richard C. "Linear Genetics, Non-Linear Epigenetics: Complementary Approaches to Understanding Complex Diseases." *Integrative Psychological and Behavioral Science* 30, no. 4 (September 1995): 273–282.

Yates, F. Eugene. "Homeokinetics/Homeodynamics: A Physical Heuristic for Life and Complexity." University of California–Los Angeles, Department of Medicine, *Ecological Psychology* 20, no. 2 (April 2008): 148–179.

Zilbut, Joseph P. "Is Physiology the Locus of Health/Health Promotion?" *Advan. Physiol. Edu.* 32 (2008): 118–119. doi: 10.1152/advan.90134.2008.

CHAPTER 4

Antonelli, Jodi, et al. "Exercise and Prostate Cancer Risk in a Cohort of Veterans Undergoing Prostate Needle Biopsy." *The Journal of Urology* 182, no. 5 (November 2009): 2101–2102.

Aubrey, Allison. "Even a Little Exercise Boosts Fitness, Study Shows." NPR, May 15, 2007. http://www.npr.org/templates/story/story.php?storyId=10192772.

Blair, Steven N., et al. "Cardiorespiratory Fitness as a Predictor of Fatal and Nonfatal Stroke in Asymptomatic Women and Men." *American Heart Association.* Stroke. 2008;39:2950–2957. http://stroke.ahajournals.org/cgi/content/abstract/39/11/2950

Bode, F. R., et al. "Age and Sex Differences in Lung Elasticity." *J. Appl. Physiol.* 41 (1976): 129–135.

Burroughs, John. *The Breath of Life* (New York: Houghton Mifflin, 1915). "Coffee, Exercise, Fight Prostate Cancer." Reporting on Harvard School of Public Health Study. (December 8, 2009) http://www.nlm.nih.gov/medlineplus/news/fullstory_92761.html

Dole, Malcolm. "The Natural History of Oxygen." *The Journal of General Physiology,* September 1, 1965.

Framingham Heart Study: A Project of the National Heart, Lung and Blood Institute and Boston University. http://www.framinghamheartstudy.org.

Importance of Aerobic Fitness: Aerobic Fitness Information. http://www.aerobictest.com/AerobicFitnessImportance.htm.

Lane, Nick. *Oxygen: The Molecule That Made the World* (New York: Oxford University Press, 2003).

Marinello, Sal. "The Health and Fitness Advice Ramble: Exercise and Cancer, ANTM Scam, Vitamin D and More." May 28, 2008. http://www.intersportswire.com/archives/235.

Martinez, Maria Elena, et al. *Colon Cancer and Exercise.* American Cancer Society, July 20, 1999. http://www.cancer.org/docroot/NWS/content/NWS_1_1x_Colon_Cancer_and_Exercise.asp.

Thyfault, John, et al. "Fatty Liver Disease, Next Big Problem for Obese and Inactive People." *Journal of Physiology* (forthcoming).

CHAPTER 5

Carmina, E., et al. "Correlates of Increased Lean Muscle Mass in Women with Polycystic Ovary Syndrome." *European Journal of Endocrinology* 161, no. 4 (July 2009): 583–589.

Ebben, William P., and Randall L. Jensen. "Strength Training for Women: Debunking Myths That Block Opportunity." *The Physician and Sports Medicine* 26, no. 5 (May 1998).

Editors Prevention Health Books for Women. *Fit Not Fat at Forty Plus: The Shape Up Plan That Balances Your Hormones, Boosts Your Metabolism, and Fights Female Fat in Your Forties— And Beyond* (Rodale Press, 2002).

Hobson, Katherine. "How to Avoid Losing Muscle As You Age." *U.S. News & World Report,* September 4, 2008. http://www.usnews.com/health/blogs/on-fitness/2008/09/04/how-to-avoid-losing-muscle-as-you-age.html.

Kenny, Anne M., et al. "Prevalence of Sarcopenia and Predictors of Skeletal Muscle Mass in Nonobese Women Who Are Long-Term Users of Estrogen-Replacement Therapy." *The Journals of Gerontology Series A: Biological Sciences and Medical Sciences* 58 (2003): M436–M440.

Magaziner J., W. Hawkes, J. R. Hebel, S. I. Zimerman, K. M. Fox, M. Dolan, et al. "Recovery from Hip Fracture in Eight Areas of Function." *Journal of Gerontology: Medical Sciences* 55A, no. 9 (2000): M498–M507.

Misner, Bill. "Interventions for Enhancing Lean Muscle Mass Gain and Fat Mass Loss During Strength or Speed Training Protocols." *AFPA Fitness,* Newsletter of the American Fitness Professionals Association, 2009.

National Center for Health Statistics. "Trends in Health and Aging." http://www.cdc .gov/nchs/agingact.htm.

Pocock, N., et al. "Muscle Strength, Physical Fitness, and Weight but Not Age Predict Femoral Neck Bone Mass." *J. Bone Miner. Res.* 4, no. 3 (June 1989): 441–448.

Poehlman, E.T., et al. "Effects of Endurance and Resistance Training on Total Daily Energy Expenditure in Young Women: A Controlled Randomized Trial." *Journal of Clinical Endocrinology and Metabolism* 87 (2002): 1004–1009.

South Dakota State University. "Lean Mass Better for Developing Bones in Young People." *ScienceDaily,* June 29, 2009. http://www.sciencedaily.com/releases/2009/ 06/090622201612.htm.

University of Alberta. "Lean Muscle Mass Helps Even Obese Patients Battle Cancer." *ScienceDaily,* December 18, 2008. http://www.sciencedaily.com_/releases/2008/ 12/081217124424.htm?utm_source=feedburner&utm_medium=feed&utm_ca mpaign=Feed%3A+sciencedaily+%28ScienceDaily.

Wang, Z., S. Heshka, K. Zhang, C. N. Boozer, and S. B. Heymsfield. "Resting Energy Expenditure: Systematic Organization and Critique of Prediction Methods." *Obesity Research* 9 (2001): 331–336.

Wright, Vonda, and Ruth Winter. *Fitness After 40: How to Stay Strong at Any Age* (AMA-COM, 2009).

Note: A good summary of facts about metabolism and metabolic rates can be found online at: http://www.healthreserve.com/dieting/metabolism.htm.

CHAPTER 6

Anecdotal centenarian profiles http://www.aolhealth.com/healthy-living/aging-well/ centenarian. Additional centenarian profiles http://www.americanprofile.com/ article/35516.html.

Bordeaux University study results on marriage and Alzheimer's disease reported in "Study Shows that Socializing Can Extend Your Life." MedicineNet.com. http://www.medicinenet.com/script/main/art.asp?articlekey=50788

Dello Buono, Marirosa, et al. "Quality of Life and Longevity: A Study of Centenarians." *Age Ageing* 27 (March 1998): 207–216.

Dychtwald, Ken. *Healthy Aging: Challenges and Solutions* (Aspen Publishing, 1999).

Fragniere, Alexandra, et al. "Using Animal Models to Investigate the Functions of Adult Hippocampal Neurogenesis." Infoscience: Le Portal D'Information Sci-entfique, 2008.

Georgia Centenarian Study. Summary http://qa.genetics.uga.edu/outlineDetails.html. Much like the New England Centenarian Study, this regional-based (state of Georgia) study has been analyzing cognitively intact centenarians since 1988.

Glass, Thomas A. et al. "Population based study of social and productive activities as predictors of survival among elderly Americans." *British Medical Journal* 319 (August 21, 1999):478–483.

Griffith, Robert W., M.D. "Centenarians' Lifestyle—What Works, What Doesn't." *HealthAndAge.com,* June 18, 2004. http://www.healthandage.com/Centenarians-Lifestyle-What-Works-What-Doesnt.

Masui, Y., et al. "Do Personality Characteristics Predict Longevity? Findings from the Tokyo Centenarian Study." *AGE* 28, no. 4 (December 2006).

National Centenarian Awareness Project. "Live to 100 and Beyond." News clips on active centenarians. http://www.liveto100andbeyond.com.

The New England Centenarian Study is summarized at: http://www.bumc.bu.edu/centenarian/overview/. This ongoing study, begun in 1994, continues to provide us with valuable insights into achieving 100 healthy years. Among this study's notable contributions is the observation that "The older you get, the healthier you've been."

Perls, Thomas, et al. "Morbidity Profiles of Centenarians: Survivors, Delayers, and Es-
capers." *The Journals of Gerontology Series A: Biological Sciences and Medical Sciences* 58
(2003): M232–M237.

"Reaching 100 for Men." *The Centenarian* (UK). http://www.thecentenarian.co.uk/
reaching–100-for-men.html.

Saczynski, Jane A., et al. "The Effect of Social Engagement on Incident Dementia."
American Journal of Epidemiology 163, no. 5 (2006): 433–440. doi: 10.1093/aje/kwj061.

Sheehy, Gail. Excerpt from *Sex and the Seasoned Woman* (2006), National Centenarian
Awareness Project. http://www.adlercentenarians.org/gail_sheehy.htm.

Wilson, Robert S., Kristin R. Krueger, Liping Gu, Julia L. Bienias, Carlos F. Mendes
de Leon, and Denis A. Evans. "Neuroticism, Extraversion, and Mortality in a De-
fined Population of Older Persons." *Psychosomatic Medicine* 67 (2005): 841–845.

Yong, Ed. "Secrets of the Centenarians: Life Begins at 100." *New Scientist,* September
7, 2009.

A summary of the findings of the value of social interaction on longevity from the
New England Centenarian Study and the Centenarian Sibling Pair Study from
researchers Margery Hutter Silver and Thomas Perls http://www.webmd.com/
healthy-aging/guide/20061101/you-too-could-live-to–100-at-least–80.

CHAPTER 7

Abramov, Leon A. "Sexual Life and Sexual Frigidity Among Women Developing
Acute Myocardial Infarction." *Psychosomatic Medicine* 38, no. 6 (November–December 1976).

Bacon, Constance G., et al. "Sexual Function in Men Older Than 50 Years of Age:
Results from the Health Professionals Follow-up Study." *Annals of Internal Medicine*

139, no. 3 (August 2003): 161–168. This study established the direct correlation between physical fitness and sexual fitness in men over 50 years of age. Callaway, Ewen. "Viagra Could Boost Orgasms in Depressed Women." *New Scientist,* July 22, 2008.

"Can Good Sex Keep You Young?" *WebMD,* November 13, 2000. http://www.webmd .com/healthy-aging/features/sex-keep-young Chalker, Rebecca. "Strategies for Staying Sexual After Menopause." *The Women's Health Activist,* May 4, 2009. http://nsrc.sfsu.edu/article/strategies_staying_sexual_after_menopause.

Davison, Sonia Louise, et al. "The Relationship between Self-Reported Sexual Satisfaction and General Well-Being in Women" *The Journal of Sexual Medicine.* 6 (10): 2690–2697.

Dubin, Charles. "Aging and Female Sexual Desire." *Smart Now.* http://www.smart-now.com/page/7882.

Esposito, Katherine, et al. "Hyperlipidemia and Sexual Function in Premenopausal Women." *Journal of Sexual Medicine* 6, no. 6 (April 23, 2009): 1696–1703. doi: 10.1111/j.1743–6109.2009.01284.x.

Geddes. Linda. "No Sex Tonight Honey, I Haven't Taken My Statins." *New Scientist,* September 8, 2009. http://www.newscientist.com/article/dn17750-no-sex-tonight-honey-i-havent-taken-my-statins.html.

Hellstrom, Wayne J. G. "Testosterone Replacement Therapy." *Digital Urology Journal* (forthcoming).

Kaufman, Miriam, Cory Silverberg, and Fran Odette. *The Ultimate Guide to Sex and Disability: For All of Us Who Live with Disabilities, Chronic Pain and Illness* (Cleis Press, 2003).

Manton, K. G. et al. "Active Life Expectancy in the U.S. Elderly Population 1982–1991: Dynamic Equilibria of Mortality and Disability." *Center for Demographic Studies.* (1993).

Marshall, Michael. "Six Things Science Has Revealed About the Female Orgasm." *New Scientist,* May 28, 2009.

Scott, Elizabeth. "Sex and Stress—The Links Between Sex and Stress." About.com Stress Management, November 24, 2008. http://stress.about.com/.

Scottish study on sex and youthful appearance cited in: BBC World News. October 10, 2000. http://news.bbc.co.uk/2/hi/uk_news/scotland/965045.stm

Smith, George Davey, et al. "Sex and Death: Are They Related? Findings from the Caerphilly Cohort Study." *BMJ* 315 (December 20, 1997): 1641–1644. This is the much-cited Welsh study showing a 50 percent decrease in mortality among men with higher orgasmic frequency.

Veronelli, Annamaria, et al. "Sexual Dysfunction Is Frequent in Premenopausal Women with Diabetes, Obesity, and Hypothyroidism, and Correlates with Markers of Increased Cardiovascular Risk. A Preliminary Report." *Journal of Sexual Medicine* 6, no. 6 (April 23, 2009): 1561–1568. doi: 10.1111/j.1743–6109.2009 .01242.x.

"Women's Sexual Activity in Later Years Influenced by Partner Issues, UCSF Study Shows." News release, University of California, San Francisco, June 24, 2009. http://news.ucsf.edu/releases/womens-sexual-activity-in-later-years-influenced-by-partner-issues-ucsf-stu/.

CHAPTER 8

Bullitt, Elizabeth, et al. "Aerobic Activity May Keep the Brain Young." *UNC Health Care Bulletin,* June 29, 2009. This bulletin reports on research to be published in *American Journal of Neuroradiology* and on research presented to the annual meeting of the Radiological Society of North America in 2008.

Castelli, D. M., et al. "Physical fitness and academic achievement in third- and fifth-grade students" *J Sport Exerc Psychol.* (2), (April 29 2007): 239–52.

Chen, H. "Physical activity and the risk of Parkinson disease." *NEUROLOGY* 64 (2005): 664–669 (Harvard University study on exercise and risk of Parkinson's disease).

"Coffee 'May Reverse' Alzheimer's." *BBC News Report.* http://news.bbc.co.uk/2/hi/health/8132122.stm.

Collihan, Kelly. "Exercise Amps Up Alzheimer's Brain?" *WebMD.com.* To be published in *Neurology* by Jeffrey M. Burns, et al. http://www.webmd.com/alzheimers/news/20080714/exercise-amps-up-alzheimers-brain.

Coughlan, Andy. "New Look at Alzheimer's Could Revolutionise Treatment." *New Scientist,* September 9, 2009.

Facklemann, Kathleen. "Research Shows Exercise Protects Against Parkinson's." *USA Today,* January 17, 2006.

Gould, Elizabeth, and Charles G. Gross. "Neurogenesis in Adult Mammals: Some Progress and Problems." *The Journal of Neuroscience* 22, no. 3 (February 1, 2002): 619–623.

Healthy Eating Pyramid. *Harvard School of Public Health.* http://www.hsph.harvard.edu/nutritionsource/what-should-you-eat/pyramid/

Hitti, Hitti. "Exercise May Help Prevent Parkinson's." *WebMD Health News,* April 23, 2007. http://www.webmd.com/parkinsons-disease/news/20070423/exercise-may-help-prevent-parkinsons.

Lund, Angela. "Preventing Alzheimer's: Exercise Still Best." *MayoClinic.com,* March 25, 2008. http://www.mayoclinic.com/health/alzheimers/MY00002.

Nelson, Bernard P. "Aerobic Exercise Effects on the Human Brain." Beckman Institute Study of Aerobics vs. Brain. *Suite101.com.* http://aerobicconditioning.suite101.com/article.cfm/beckman_institute_study_of_aerobics_vs_brain.

Paddock, Catherine. "Being Overweight Linked to 'Severe Brain Degeneration.'" *MedicalNewsToday.com,* August 27, 2009. http://www.medicalnewstoday.com/articles/162135.php.

Patoine, Brenda. "Move Your Feet, Grow New Neurons? Exercise Induced Neurogenesis Shown in Humans." *The Dana Review.* (May 01, 2007). A report on human neurogenesis research at Columbia University. http://www.dnalc.org/view/848-Exercise-induced-Neurogenesis.html.

Ratey, John J. *Spark: The Revolutionary New Science of Exercise and the Brain* (New York: Little, Brown, 2008).

Rayl, A. J. S. "Research Turns Another "Fact" Into Myth." *The Scientist* 13(4) (1999):16 http://www.the-scientist.com/article/display/18407/

"Research Shows Exercise Protects Against Parkinson's." Parkinson's Disease Foundation, *Science News.* (Jan. 17, 2006) (Report on University of Pittsburgh research study)

Richardson, Vanessa. "A Fit Body Means a Fit Mind." *Edutopia.* http://www.edutopia.org/exercise-fitness-brain-benefits-learning#.

Rodrigue, Raz N. "Differential Aging of the Brain: Patterns, Cognitive Correlates and Modifiers." *Neurosci. Biobehav. Rev.* 30, no. 6 (2006): 730–748. http://www.ncbi.nlm.nih.gov/pubmed/16919333.

Scarmeas, Richard, et al. "Physical Activity, Diet, and Risk of Alzheimer Disease." *JAMA* 302(6) (2009):627–637.

Schnabel, Jim. "Physical Fitness Linked to Larger Hippocampus in Elderly." *The Dana Foundation Newsletter,* (April 2009). Reporting on a University of Illinois study on exercise and brain growth in the elderly. http://www.dana.org/news/features/detail.aspx?id=21078

Shors, Tracy J. "How to Save New Brain Cells." *Scientific American,* March 2009. http://www.scientificamerican.com/article.cfm?id=saving-new-brain-cells.   Shultz,

Nora. "Expanding Waistlines May Cause Shrinking Brains." *New Scientist,* August 23, 2009.

Vaynman, S., Z. Ying, and F. Gomez-Pinilla. "Hippocampal BDNF Mediates the Efficacy of Exercise on Synaptic Plasticity and Cognition." *Eur. J. Neurosci.* 20, no. 10 (November 2004): 2580–2590.

CHAPTER 9

About Herbs, Botanicals & Other Products. Memorial Sloan-Kettering Cancer Center. http://www.mskcc.org/mskcc/html/11570.cfm. This online information resource, compiled and maintained by the Integrative Medicine Service of Sloan-Kettering, provides evidence-based information about herbs, botanicals, supplements, and more. This remarkable compilation of scientific information about everything from antioxidants to acupuncture to vitamins is an exceptional resource.

Albanese, Emiliano, et al. "Dietary Fish and Meat Intake and Dementia in Latin America, China, and India: A 10/66 Dementia Research Group Population-Based Study." *American Journal of Clinical Nutrition* 90, no. 2 (August 2009): 392–400.

Bjelakovic, Goran, et al. "Mortality in Randomized Trials of Antioxidant Supplements for Primary and Secondary Preventio." *JAMA* 297 (2007):842–857.

Bortz, Walter M., et al. "The Effect of Feeding Frequency on Rate of Weight Loss." *New England Journal of Medicine* 274 (1966): 376–379.

Centenarian Study Booklet. Georgia Centenarian Study. http://www.geron.uga.edu/pdfs/CentStudyBooklet.pdf.

"Coenzyme Q10." National Cancer Institute, U.S. National Institutes of Health. A summary of studies on the use of Coenzyme Q10 in cancer treatment. http://www.cancer.gov/cancertopics/pdq/cam/coenzymeQ10/Patient

ConsumerLab.com. http://www.consumerlab.com/. A consumer information source based on independent testing of commercially available vitamins, supplements, herbal remedies, etc. Manufacturers' claims are tested and reported on.

"Death Link to Too Much Red Meat." *BBC World News,* March 24, 2009. http://news.bbc.co.uk/2/hi/health/7959128.stm.

DeKosky, Steven T., et al. "*Ginkgo biloba* for Prevention of Dementia." *JAMA* 300(19) (2008):2253–2262.

Evans, Martin. "Tips for a Longer Life According to the World's Oldest People." *The Daily Telegraph* (UK), November 26, 2009. http://www.telegraph.co.uk/news/6652291/Tips-for-a-longer-life-according-to-the-worlds-oldest-people.html.

"Food Pyramids: What Should You Really Eat?" Harvard School of Public Health, Cambridge, MA. http://www.hsph.harvard.edu/nutritionsource/what-should-you-eat/pyramid/.

Heaney, Mark L., et al. "Vitamin C Antagonizes the Cytotoxic Effects of Antineoplastic Drugs." *Cancer Research* 68 (October 1, 2008): 8031.

Herbal Information: Dietary Supplements; Food and Nutrition Information Center. U.S. Department of Agriculture, National Agricultural Library.

Hooper, M., and R. Heighway-Bury. *Who Built the Pyramid?* (Cambridge, MA: Candlewick Press, 2001).

Misner, Bill. "Interventions for Enhancing Lean Muscle Mass Gain and Fat Mass Loss During Strength or Speed Training Protocols." American Fitness Professionals Association. http://www.afpafitness.com/articles/articles-and-newletters/

research-articles-index/exercise-program-design/interventions-for-enhancing-lean-muscle-mass-gain-and-fat-mass-loss-during-strength-or-speed-training-protocols–2/.

"Overweight Top World's Hungry." *BBC World News,* August 15, 2006. http://news .bbc.co.uk/2/hi/health/4793455.stm. Parker-Pop, Tara. "Vitamins, a False Hope?" *New York Times,* February 16, 2009. http://www.nytimes.com/2009/02/17/health/ 17well.html?_r=2.

Pollan, Michael. *In Defense of Food: An Eater's Manifesto* (New York: Penguin, 2008).

"Putting Limits on Vitamin E: The Potent Antioxidant May Do More Harm Than Good." Unpublished report from Tel Aviv University. http://www.physorg.com/ news181403527.html.

"Scientists Find Molecular Trigger That Helps Prevent Aging and Disease." *Science Daily,* (November 23, 2009). http://www.sciencedaily.com/releases/2009/11/091 118143217.htm

Stibich, Mark. "Turmeric: Anti-Aging Miracle Spice?" *About.com Guide,* August 31, 2008. http://longevity.about.com/od/antiagingfoods/a/turmeric.htm.

"Tomato Pill 'Beats Heart Disease.'" *BBC World News,* June 1, 2009. http://news.bbc .co.uk/2/hi/health/8076556.stm.

Trivedi, Bijal. "The Calorie Delusion: Why Food Labels Are Wrong." *New Scientist,* July 15, 2009. http://www.newscientist.com/article/mg20327171.200-the-calorie-delusion.html?DCMP=NLC-nletter&nsref=mg20327171.200.

"Typical Lifetime Dietary Habits of Centenarians." *The Centenarian* (UK). http:// www.thecentenarian.co.uk/typical-lifetime-dietary-habits-of-centenarians.html. A survey of dietary characteristics of notable centenarian populations, including Azerbaijan, Sardinia, Okinawa, etc.

University of Michigan Food Pyramid. http://www.med.umich.edu/umim/food-pyramid/.

U.S. Department of Agriculture, Center for Nutrition Policy and Promotion. *The Healthy Eating Index.* 1995.

"Vitamin E." National Institutes of Health, Office of Dietary Supplements. http://ods.od.nih.gov/factsheets/VitaminE.asp. Includes results of numerous vitamin-specific studies relating to heart disease and cancer.

"Weekly Curry May Fight Dementia." *BBC World News,* June 3, 2009. http://news.bbc.co.uk/2/hi/health/8080630.stm.

Women's Health Initiative. *Findings.* http://www.whi.org/findings/

CHAPTER 10

Bortz, Walter M. *Next Medicine: The Science and Civics of Health* (New York: Oxford University Press, 2010).

Csikszentmihalyi, Mihaly. *Flow: The Psychology of Optimal Experience.* (New York: Harper Perennial Modern Classics, 2008).

EPILOGUE

Yalom, Irvin D. *Staring at the Sun: Overcoming the Terror of Death* (Berkeley: Jossey-Bass, 2009).

INDEX